Quick and Simple Chair Yoga for Seniors Over 60

The Fully Illustrated Guide to Seated Poses and
Cardio Exercises for Weight Loss and Mobility to
Maintain Your Independence in
Under 10 Minutes a day!

Audrey Fitzgerald

First edition, 2022.

www.gesundbooks.com

~Dedications~

To my dear father who was such a wonderful provider in so many ways and who left such an amazing legacy for us to follow.

To my dear mother who taught me by example to march to the beat of my own drum and is such an inspiration of living well in her golden years.

To my awesome brother who was always so supportive of me and a great, encouraging influence in my life since childhood.

Table of Contents

A FREE GIFT TO ALL MY READERS!

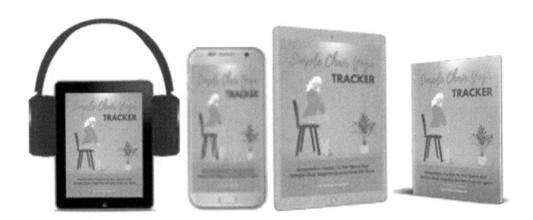

Dear Friends,

As a thank you and to help you stay dedicated to stick to your chair yoga and exercise goals, I would like to send you a free copy of my colorful 30-day simple chair yoga tracker so you can track your progress at home and keep your motivation alive!

To get your free copy now, please visit:

www.gesundbooks.com

Introduction

The secret of getting ahead is getting started. –Mark Twain

Do you find yourself struggling to do things that you used to do with ease? Is reaching for things on the top shelf or climbing the stairs becoming a little more difficult? Do you struggle with eliminating stubborn fat buildup? If you answered yes to these questions, you're not alone, so don't despair! There's plenty you can do to regain lost muscle tone without disrupting your daily routine, and the rewards of exercise are plentiful. If you are here to prevent these situations from happening, you are also in the right place. Either way, I am very excited for you that you have chosen this journey!

Staying active is key to good health and overall well-being. It is even more important for older adults because it helps impede age-related challenges. Innumerable studies prove the important health benefits of physical activity and exercise for seniors. Regular physical exercise helps improve your mental health. Studies indicate that regular body movement enhances the secretion of "feel good" hormones known as endorphins. These hormones help relieve stress, make you feel happy, and give you a sense of well-being throughout your life (Domonell, 2016).

Maintaining regular physical exercise is also helpful in chronic disease prevention. Studies indicate that staying physically active helps boost your immunity and prevent common chronic illnesses (Gopinath et al., 2018). The health benefits of physical activity and exercise for seniors are endless: bone loss prevention, relieves osteoarthritis pain, improved body strength, flexibility, balance and coordination, reduced risk of falls, improved sleep, and more.

While exercises like strength training and high-intensity workouts are effective and build body strength, they can be a little harder for seniors and people with mobility problems. It also could be a bit difficult for seniors to get incentivized to want to go for a long run or gym session. You may want to get up and move but feel fatigued and lethargic. The good news is that you don't need to be a fitness fanatic in order to reap the benefits of physical exercise. Even a light exercise or movement can be powerful. So if you've never been a big exercise fan, don't worry.

As we age, we can feel that we don't have the necessary support system to be consistent with exercise or enjoy the experience. Don't lose hope. It is never too late. There are several things you can do to offset "Mother Nature." This book has got you covered.

Whether you're tired of waking up sore and achy or just want to get moving in a fun, new way, you've found the right book for you. It is the best solution to all your age-related and fitness woes. By following the teachings inside, you will move better, feel better, be more productive, and have more energy, awareness, and joy! In this book, you will learn:

Simple, accessible exercises that can be done at home even after injuries or with limited mobility.

- The benefits of a yoga practice and exercise routine.

- The basics of stretching for flexibility

- Poses geared toward weight loss.

- A quick and simple yoga and cardio routine that can be done in under 10 minutes.

- Diet recommendations for increasing flexibility and decreasing inflammation.

- The power of mindset, positivity, and optimism to the body

With this newfound knowledge, you'll find yourself approaching exercise with confidence and ease and enjoying the experience all along the way. You'll find relief from your bodily aches and pains and feel more flexible and active. You'll learn how to harness the power of your mind to experience a richer, more fulfilled life while boosting the numerous health benefits of exercise.

I have taken my mom through yoga routines, advised her on what to include in her diet for the past 20 years, and watched her experience all these benefits. I have been interested in fitness and well-being since I was a teenager, and in 1996, I trained as a professional chef. I began making healthy alternatives to the recipes I was learning and founded a natural foods personal chef and catering company that focused on overall client wellness. In 2001, I started studying alignment-based yoga and became a yoga, meditation, and movement teacher. I then founded a wellness lifestyle coaching company that focused on a body-mind-spirit approach to well-being. It is now two decades down the line, and I still love sharing yoga and nutritional advice with loved ones!

My mom just turned 80, and at the time of this writing, she plays ping pong five days a week. She loves moving her body while having fun with friends! When I was in my late twenties, I started teaching her yoga, and she was in her early sixties. I would teach her poses to do when she was on her own. In the beginning, it wasn't easy for her, but after giving her the tricks and information I am sharing in this book, everything fell into place, and I believe she achieved the promised end results. I really think that this ongoing yoga over the course of 20 years has a lot to do with her ability to still play ping pong at age 80! I wish that type of mobility for all seniors, and that's why I'm writing this book.

I share this story just to inspire people, but I really feel like beginning yoga at any age will be helpful to your health journey! So even if you have no prior yoga experience or no prior exercise experience, start today, and you will benefit!

I hope this book will empower you to remain fit and active and feel your best as you approach your golden years. If I was able to teach my mom yoga at age 60 and she still practices it to prevent pain at age 80, I believe that you, too, will be able to find the same relief from your aches and pains. I want you to be empowered to live your optimal life through a healthy lifestyle. I am passionate about sharing healthy strategies and modalities with people, and I want to help as many people as possible!

Chapter 1:

Why Yoga?

I feel so lucky to have discovered yoga and to have fully integrated it into my life's rhythm. Not only has the practice helped me physically, but it has also taught me the discipline of having a consistent morning routine that prepares me emotionally and physically for the day ahead. Discovering the unexpected benefits of yoga made it clear to me that not enough people know about all the rewards of this practice!

In this chapter, I am going to discuss scientifically proven health benefits of yoga practice, why chair yoga is an excellent option for seniors, common myths about yoga, and how to approach overall wellness.

The Benefits of Yoga

Yoga is more than just a physical form of exercise—it's a spiritual, mindful practice with a host of benefits. Originating thousands of years ago in ancient India, this practice began as a philosophical framework that is sometimes forgotten in Western practices. In the past few decades, research on yoga has massively increased, and there are dozens of empirical studies confirming the beneficial effects of yoga on physical and mental health. If you have never tried yoga before, here are some incentives to do so!

- Reduced stress and depression: Studies indicate that yoga practice can help decrease the symptoms of depression, stress, and anxiety in anybody, including seniors above 60 (Bridges & Sharma, 2017). Research also proves that regular body movement, including yoga, tells your body to release endorphins, the "feel good" hormones relieving stress, leaving you happy, composed, and satisfied (Domonell, 2016). In addition to this, any yoga practice inherently requires you to be mindful of your breathing and includes meditative movements. This enables you to shift your focus from stressful thoughts to the present, thus promoting peace and relaxation.

- Weight loss: Yoga is not only good for busting stress but is also, surprisingly, one of the most effective regimens for weight loss. Yes, yoga is very efficacious in eliminating stubborn fat buildup. Yoga is a form of physical activity, and as discussed earlier, exercise enhances the secretion of "feel good" hormones (endorphins). These hormones dominate the stress-causing hormone (cortisol, which, in turn, increases insulin sensitivity. This helps improve your metabolism, thus enhancing nutrient partitioning—"telling" your body to burn up food and use it as energy to fuel your body instead of storing it as fat (Bird & Hawley, 2017). When practiced regularly, yoga can help you shed some pounds and cut down on weight.

- Improved respiration: The breathing exercises and the breath control practices in yoga help to expand your lung capacity as well as increasing oxygen flow, thus improving your pulmonary health. One study conducted on elderly women to determine the influence of yoga on pulmonary function found that those who took a 12-week yoga program and remained consistent throughout this period experienced significant improvement in their pulmonary function (Bezera et al., 2014).

- Improved sleep: We all know that adequate sleep is a key and essential element of a person's well-being. Your energy levels, cellular structures, and memory are all repaired and restored during sleep. If you struggle with getting enough sleep at night, get hooked on a yoga program. Yoga practice can help regulate your body's circadian rhythm and improve your sleep quality during the night. It provides just the right amount of exertion without pushing you to the point of discomfort or getting you exhausted. To back this up, a recent study conducted on the effectiveness of yoga on sleep quality demonstrated that yoga intervention is effective in managing insomnia and other sleep problems (Wang et al., 2020).

- Enhanced balance, flexibility, mobility, and stability: You already know that flexibility and balance are key in performing daily tasks and for independence and movement. Seniors who practice yoga enjoy improved mobility and stability. This is especially true for those who practice chair yoga because a properly done chair yoga routine places emphasis on feet and joints, stretching and strengthening them. The breathing techniques (holding a pose for several breaths) during the practice also help relax and loosen your muscles and connective tissues, increasing your range of motion. One study published in the international journal of therapy proves that practicing chair yoga can dramatically boost the overall flexibility of older adults (Ferinatti et al., 2014).

- Chronic disease management: Yoga enhances positive effects on many chronic diseases. It is also a preventative measure against lifestyle-related diseases caused by a sedentary lifestyle, overeating, being overweight, or alcohol/tobacco consumption. For instance, seniors with type 2 diabetes may ease, prevent, or control its effects by performing light yoga poses or stretches that benefit the pancreas. Like any other physical activity, yoga practice regulates insulin production as well as massaging your internal organs. This, in turn, improves your cholesterol and glucose levels. Yoga is also known for blood pressure reduction. Seniors who practice yoga experience lower blood pressure after their first yoga class and maintain it when they stay consistent. So if you battle hypertension, this is a great way to get rid of it. According to The Centers for Disease Control and Prevention reports, seniors who stay physically active by performing regular exercises have lower rates of stroke, coronary heart disease, hypertension, and many other chronic diseases (Older Adults, 1999).

- Strengthened bones: If you are worried about brittle bones and osteoarthritis, try yoga! Seniors who practice yoga have reported increased bone and body strength. Regular yoga practice can help boost your bone strength. A promising study in postmenopausal women indicated that yoga improves bone density (Harvard Health, (2022)). Strong bones make you flexible and less prone to falls.

- Improved mental health: Yoga practice enhances mindfulness, resilience, happiness, well-being, life satisfaction, and social relationships.

- Increased mind-body connection: Yoga cultivates a mind-body connection creating a better harmony between your body, mind, and spirit. It teaches us to develop a mindset that helps us to approach challenges from a place of soul-searching, excitement, and exploration.

Why Chair Yoga?

Anybody can practice yoga and reap all of the above benefits. However, due to the different levels of difficulty and an intricate repertoire of ancient yoga, practicing traditional yoga can be daunting to those who are new to the idea, people who want to start slowly, those who are not steady on their feet, or those who would just feel more confident sitting down. This is especially true for people with mobility problems.

While yoga is more accessible for seniors than many believe, chair yoga creates the perfect approach that is accessible for everyone regardless of weight, age, shape, gender, disabilities, chronic conditions, previous injuries, or level of experience. In other words, anyone can practice chair yoga, including those who just want to increase his or her range of motion through gradual and gentle exercises.

Chair yoga is a type of yoga from the Hatha branch of yoga. Hatha is the yoga of the body that includes poses, breathing, and meditation. Chair yoga can be done either sitting for the entire session or, in some classes, standing and using the chair as a prop for balance. Seniors can enjoy all the benefits of regular yoga without having to get up and down off of the floor or stressing their joints.

Biggest Yoga Myths

There is a lot of information about yoga on the internet, most of which is unproven. With access to today's technology information, most people who decide to embark on their yoga practice journey get advice on how to do it by digging through the internet for the poses because it is the fastest source. Unfortunately, many fitness blogs, social media posts, and other internet sources perpetuate many yoga myths.

For instance, if you try searching for yoga poses on Instagram accounts, you are likely to be bombarded with young, slim, flexible females pulling off perfect-looking poses. This immediately creates the perception that yoga is only meant for young, slim, and flexible females. This causes many people to miss out on the plethora of benefits that comes with practicing yoga!

That's why I decided to debunk some of the most common myths and misconceptions about yoga that may keep you away. Read on!

1. **You must be flexible to practice yoga.** You don't have to be flexible in order to begin your yoga practice. Just start from where you are, and with time, you will become more flexible. The purpose of performing yoga is to improve your physical situation, not to become a "pro" or show off. As discussed earlier, yoga practice helps improve flexibility; the more you stay consistent with your yoga classes, the more you become flexible. It doesn't have to be complicated poses. Even just a few minutes of dynamic stretches are sufficient to improve your flexibility. One study conducted on male athletes showed that men who completed 10 weeks of yoga with only 2 classes per week experienced increased flexibility and mobility in their hamstring muscles, lower back, ankle, hip, and shoulder joints (Polsgrove et al., 2016). So, don't let unreasonable yoga myths like this one hold you back from giving it a try!

2. **Yoga is nothing more than stretching and balancing.** Yoga is comprehensive and involves much more than a normal physical practice. Besides engaging with the physical body, yoga encourages you to focus on your mind and inner self. This helps cultivate a connection with yourself, creating a better

harmony between your body, mind, and spirit. It helps you know how your body feels from the inside and be able to make wise decisions as far as your system is concerned.

3. **Only younger people can practice yoga.** Yoga is for everyone, regardless of your age and gender. In fact, older people need yoga even more. You are likely to benefit more from yoga if you are older than the young people. Of course, just like any other physical activity, it is important for older adults to take precautions while practicing yoga to prevent injuries. The good thing with yoga is that you can simply adapt the postures, no matter how stiff your body is. Thanks to chair yoga, you can easily improve flexibility and body strength by practicing yoga regularly, no matter your physical limitations. There are so many advantages of yoga that make it an excellent choice for the elderly. For instance, some yoga poses, like the tree pose, helps older adults who struggle with balance and flexibility to improve. A study conducted on women of different age groups showed that women who completed 20 weeks of Hatha yoga sessions with only 1 session per week experienced increased mobility and flexibility of their spine and hamstring muscles as well as increased range of motion in the joints, irrespective of their age (Grabara & Szopa, 2015).

4. **You have to be slim to do yoga.** Fitness centers and yoga studios often show slim people performing complex twists when advertising their yoga classes and programs. This creates the assumption that yoga classes are only good for slim and flexible people. However, this isn't true. In fact, research shows that yoga can actually help with body image. One study conducted on a group of young adults who were followed for more than 15 years showed that practicing yoga promotes higher levels of body satisfaction (Neumark-Sztainer et al., 2018). Yoga can be done by anyone, regardless of your body size, shape, or fitness level! The wisdom of yoga is that the poses are there to benefit you. Most yoga poses can be adapted with the use of props like blocks, straps, or bolsters—making it easier for anyone to perform them.

5. **Yoga is just for women.** If you follow the history of yoga, you will find that it used to be taught as a "workout" to young boys by a Prince in India back in the early 1800s. But in current times, it can seem like women have taken over yoga! This misconception arises from the stereotypes people see, hear, or read. For instance, when people search for the most popular yoga social media accounts, they are likely to be flooded with images of slim, super flexible women pulling off difficult twists. This myth also arises due to the fact that women are naturally more flexible than men. However, you need to understand that flexibility is not

a requirement to begin yoga practice. Instead, it is something that you develop through yoga practice. And anybody can enjoy the benefits of yoga regardless of gender.

6. **Yoga belongs to one religion.** Yoga has been tied to Hinduism, Buddhism, and Jainism since its origin in India more than 4,000 years ago. It first featured in a collection of Hindu scriptures known as "Upanishads." This collection of over 200 scriptures described several meditation techniques to help people discover their truest selves. Yoga was also practiced by the Hindus in order to help their people achieve inner peace. However, it was not considered religious. Unlike religion, yoga practice doesn't require the worship of any deities, a formal set of rituals, or obligations. So if you are religious, don't let myths such as this one prevent you from enjoying the amazing benefits of yoga. In fact, the meditative aspect of yoga offers you the opportunity to strengthen your own faith due to the stillness, attention, and self-reflection that comes with it. Therefore, you can use yoga to connect with any higher power you believe in, or it can be a secular practice altogether.

7. **Yoga is time-consuming.** Some people prefer making their yoga sessions longer in order to dive deeper into meditation and perfect their postures, which consumes a pretty good quantity of time. This is where this yoga myth comes from. Just like any other exercise, consistency or frequency is more important than duration or the number of yoga poses done in a single day. For instance, doing a 5-minute yoga session every day for 7 days is more beneficial than doing a 2-hour session once per week. On a regular basis, it can be unrealistic to take hours for one yoga session. Besides, it is not easy to stay consistent with long yoga sessions. Shorter sessions are more sustainable because they can easily fit into your daily program. Practicing yoga in short bursts motivates you to stay consistent and form a habit. The good thing about yoga practice is that you can do it anywhere, any time. You don't have to wait for the "right" time. You can easily adapt it to your schedule and make it fit in with your lifestyle. You can even spare 5–10 minutes for yoga while waiting for your evening meal to cook!

8. **You can only practice yoga when you are completely healthy.** If you are healthy, yoga will help you maintain and improve your state. If you are not healthy, practicing yoga will help boost your immunity and manage any health condition you may be encountering. Some people believe that you shouldn't do yoga if you have asthma. On the contrary, yoga helps boost your heart and lung function. Thanks to the breathing techniques which aid the supply of enough oxygen to your lungs. Yoga also helps increase lung capacity, which enhances a

healthy breathing pattern and, thus, reducing the severity of the symptoms of asthma. Many seniors fall victim to this myth because they experience back and joint pain. They tend to believe that practicing yoga would worsen their situation, but this is not true! In fact, yoga is the most effective and cheapest remedy for back and joint pain. Several studies have proved this. One study published in the Annals of Internal Medicine shows that yoga helps ease lower back pain (Chang & Kertesz, 2017). Another study conducted to compare the effectiveness of yoga and the usual patient care for severe chronic or recurrent lower back pain proved yoga intervention as most effective because it resulted in greater improvement in back function among the participants of yoga than the normal patient care (Tilbrook et al., 2011).

9. **Yoga is dangerous.** This is one of the most common yoga myths. However, it is important to understand that any form of physical activity is only dangerous when done incorrectly. As discussed earlier, yoga has several benefits to your overall health, including increased body strength. Being weak is more dangerous than practicing yoga. You just have to ensure that you perform the poses correctly and allow your body enough time to recover in between sessions. Make sure you are carrying out all your poses in proper body form and that you are not overdoing it. Pay attention to your body and immediately stop if you feel unusual pain when doing a posture. Use simpler modifications when you feel pain. By doing so, you will avoid unnecessary injuries and reap all the benefits of yoga!

Approaching Overall Wellness

Starting and keeping up with a healthy lifestyle is a common thing to struggle with. Wellness is about more than just physical activity, although exercise plays a critical role in overall health.

What's most important about a wellness routine is making it accessible and realistic for you—setting realistic goals and developing an exercise plan that can help ensure your success in the long term. You'll also feel good as you reach your goals and make progress with your flexibility and strength.

Another critical aspect to wellness is nutrition and diet. Fueling your body in a healthful way also fuels your mind. It empowers you to tackle new challenges and experiences as you get older.

Making sure you get enough sleep is also essential. According to the National Center for Biotechnology Information, a lack of sleep can cause short-term cognitive impairment and long-term cognitive decline. Getting enough sleep, and good quality sleep at that, is linked to an increased ability to perform daily activities and overall improved mental well-being.

Stress management brings peace of mind and can improve immune function. Yoga can create physical feelings of well-being by producing endorphins and bringing you peace of mind through the spiritual aspects. There are also many poses that specifically help you to relax.

Yoga has been instrumental over the years, keeping me flexible to do the things I love. I was quite into extreme sports as a youngster and actually all the way up into my early forties. I loved surfing and skimboarding and did them every day.

Yoga was a great thing to learn early in life to keep me limber and fit for these intense activities. I credit yoga for helping me have longevity in these sports for a lot longer than most people in my age group. Many people stop doing these kinds of activities in their late twenties and early thirties.

I was even able to teach my nephew some of these sports when he was a child and was able to engage with him all the way into his teenage years. That was such a wonderful thing—to be able to bond with him in that way. I'm so grateful I had such a long run with these activities. I really believe that the flexibility and mobility I gained from doing yoga helped keep me in the game for so long and granted me that wonderful time with my nephew.

Another reason I love yoga is that I am self-employed and work from home at a desk. And taking a lot of breaks to do chair yoga right from my office chair has been integral to staying healthy, even with a more sedentary work life. Yoga taught me the discipline to practice self-care on a daily basis, and I am so thankful for that!

As mentioned, yoga is about more than just the physical aspect of exercise. Your attitude and mindset play a significant role in the level of success and satisfaction you'll gain from regular practice. Keep reading to discover more about the power of your mental attitude and its effects on you.

Chapter Two:

The Power of Mindset on the Body

Have you tried new fitness programs in the past and found yourself disappointed or frustrated? Don't worry; you are not alone! Trying new fitness programs usually comes with a couple of challenges, disappointments, and frustrations. This is especially true for beginners. This is because adaptation is a gradual process that demands a change of routine and adjusting to different ways of doing things, which can be difficult. But it is more than possible and is absolutely worth the effort! One of the first steps to achieving this is assessing your mindset and recognizing any limiting beliefs you might hold about yourself and fitness.

In this chapter, I am going to discuss the power of a healthy attitude in finding success in reaching goals. I will discuss the importance of having a growth mindset and expecting success, including strategies for developing your mindset. Let's dive in!

The Power of Having a Growth Mindset

The belief that we can triumph over challenges and obstacles that come our way is a very powerful one to have! Developing a growth mindset helps you approach challenges from a place of excitement and exploration rather than believing that you can't overcome them.

The mindset theory states that our beliefs influence the way we behave and respond to life's situations. Basically, the way you regard yourself impacts and dictates your life. It also influences how people around you will treat you. The way you view yourself will also determine your success in realizing your goals. When you sympathize with yourself, your peers and other people will treat you with the same measure of high self-esteem.

People who are attached to their basic qualities, like intelligence, athleticism, and talents, are those with fixed mindsets. And such people rarely embrace change. On the other hand, those with growth mindsets are flexible in terms of handling situations and circumstances. They believe that talents and abilities can be developed through effort and experience with time. They are usually very progressive thinkers.

Attitude is the main driving factor behind a person being in a fixed or growth mindset. This is the reason why many of us may initially hold fixed mindsets about accepting and embracing certain changes or failures—without even realizing it. Failure is not the end but an opportunity to begin again. Life is a journey of trial and error, learning and experimentation! The key is to focus on the present and enjoy the moment; doing so helps you to find yourself having an improved overall experience with yoga.

Strategies for Developing a Growth Mindset and a Positive Attitude

I want to start by saying negative emotions are not inherently bad but are a natural part of the human experience. However, if not kept under control, they can overtake your life and create a lot of problems ranging from emotional to mental to physical as well as spiritual. What we want to avoid is the unchecked rumination and repetitive thought cycles that are not only unpleasant but also very much unhelpful! Being aware of your thoughts can assist a lot with this and is important in the journey to being mindful of the content of your day-to-day mental chatter. We should make an effort to be intentional with our thoughts and gain control over our minds instead of letting the mind run wild.

On that note, below are a few different techniques by which you can train yourself to think positively and create a healthy attitude about life:

- *Smile more:* This reduces heart rate and blood pressure when one is feeling stress or anxiety. Attending fun events can help one smile. Spend time with friends who lift you up and make you feel good. Go out into nature and smile at the beautiful views! Pet the cat or the dog. Listen to pleasant music. Play with the grandkids or other fun children in your life. You can also simply sit down and watch comical movies or funny, upbeat TV shows. All of these are remedies to keep you healthy through smiling. Whether it is a good or bad day, just smile because it is a super dose of medicine to any stressful situation!

- *Practice reframing:* Change your perspective to change your mood. If something undesirable happens, look for the silver linings. You may not see them yet, but the more you look, the more you build the muscle to find them. Most people don't realize that the way your outlook is formed is actually a habit that you build, and it can either go positive or negative depending on what thoughts you habitually think. We actually have neural pathways in our brain that get formed to think a certain way, and when you learn a new way to look at things and think about things, you actually recreate these grooves in your brain! It's called neuroplasticity, and it's the brain's capability to recreate itself by forming new neural pathways and removing those pathways that are not needed any longer. It's fascinating, and we can learn a lot from it! I have actually experienced this in my life. When I was younger, my habit was to look at things negatively and respond with irrational stress and worry that was not based on logic or reality when things would go badly. Over time I told myself that this behavior was wasted energy. Then I started working on catching myself doing it and replacing those thoughts with better quality or more helpful thoughts and, eventually, my natural reaction began to change. And now, my brain starts with the more helpful, rational, logical thoughts on its own. Keep this in mind as you start your yoga journey. It's easy to get frustrated when you're new to an exercise but keep encouraging yourself and reminding yourself that Rome wasn't built in a day!

- *Build resiliency:* Your ability to feel better quickly after something unpleasant is an act of resilience. Perception is everything! Go back to the previous step of reframing to perceive your situation in a brighter light. Look at the big picture. Will this negative thing matter in 10 years? Does it matter in comparison to some greater hardships we see others go through?

- *Focus on the good things:* It is advantageous to focus on some good things if confronted with challenges and trying moments. When plans fall through, it affords you time and mental energy to do other things. Maybe it is a chance to seize a different opportunity. We don't always know what the outcome will be at the moment. In the long run, a challenging situation can turn out to be a good thing. So do not let challenges get you down. Focus on the good things you have going for yourself now and be open to your present situation turning out better in the future.

- *Practice gratitude:* Gratitude is the feeling of being grateful and wanting to express your thankfulness. Gratitude practice has been proven to reduce stress, raise self-esteem, and encourage or promote resilience during trying and complex times. Your mind, soul, and spirit can be instead occupied with thoughts, people, and things that soothe your well-being and steer you toward happiness. The mind can only truly feel one emotion at a time, so gratitude can drown out and replace stress and worry. Learn to express your gratitude to those around you, like colleagues, friends, family, and even your pets, for their unconditional love.

- *Keep a gratitude journal:* Jot down everything you hold with high esteem and gratitude. This helps in improving your optimism and sense of well-being. When passing through hard times and trying moments, peruse through your gratitude journals, and you will get refreshed and relive those happy times you once felt grateful for.

- *Laugh more:* Ever heard the saying that "laughter is the best medicine?" Laughing helps in nourishing life on a daily basis. Laughter is a strong medicine that draws people together in ways that trigger healthy, physical, and emotional changes in the body. According to the Mayo clinic, laughter strengthens your immune system, boosts mood, diminishes pain, and protects a person from the damaging effects of stress (Stress relief . . . 2021). Humor lightens burdens, inspires hope, and connects a person to others. Deep laughter can bring feelings of ecstasy and bliss. Laughter also helps you to release anger and forgive others sooner.

- *Practice positive self-talk:* Self-talk is also known as your inner voice or monologue. It usually provides that running monologue on our lives throughout the day. It is worth realizing that self-talk can be positive, motivating, cheerful, supportive, or negative and depressing. Take note of which of these inner voices you listen to, positive or negative, because positive self-talk calms and bolsters your confidence, whereas negative self-talk brings you down. A positive inner voice encourages increased feelings of happiness, self-confidence, healthy habits like a good diet and physical exercise, and decreases negative attitudes and behaviors.

- *Start each day on a high note:* There is nothing like waking up on the right side of the bed. You could start the day off with meditation, journaling, or these chair yoga exercises you are about to learn! Any of these would be a wonderful way to kick off the day. You don't need much time; even 10 minutes is a great start. What a wonderful message of love and care you give yourself right at the beginning of the day. Bonus points for doing any of these activities out in the morning sunlight!

- *Spend time with positive people:* It is paramount for us to carefully select who we spend most of our time with. Make sure that those you hang around with are adding value to your life and well-being. It has been said that you are the sum of the five people you spend the most time with. I believe this wholeheartedly and feel it is so important that I devote the whole next section to this concept and why you should choose your companions wisely. Once I learned this, it made a huge difference in my life! We are greatly influenced by those we are around, so we need to be very discerning when choosing those people—and especially so when changing our lifestyle habits! When you are working on improving exercise, diet, and mindset habits, you really want to try and find some people who are also trying to change these areas or are already very well balanced in these areas. If you don't know anyone around you who takes good care of themselves in these ways, try to find a support group in your area or a Facebook group you can join and cheer each other on as you improve your habits! As you read the next section, consider these traits to look for in friends, colleagues, and accountability buddies!

Advantages of Spending Time with Positive People

- *Positive people are guided by a healthy mindset:* They limit negativity and are quite receptive to a good life and good things. Such people help change the way you look at things and the happenings around you, improving your life mindset.

- *They are more likely to inspire you:* They help give you the desire, confidence, and enthusiasm to do something well. They see and value people's desires. They work smart and encourage others to do the same. Their way of life is an inspiration to those around them. They tend to look after their health physically, mentally, spiritually, and emotionally: They put in the work and effort toward this because they know that these four areas, if well nourished, can really make life exceptional!

- *They embrace teamwork:* As the saying goes, there is strength in unity. Positive people usually thrive in involving other people because by doing so, they achieve a lot due to joint efforts of shared experiences and expertise. Teamwork makes life easier, faster, and more efficient. Additionally, creativity is shared by all when working together, and the virtue of teamwork promotes peace, love, and unity among people who have common or shared goals.

- *They encourage better relationships with each other:* They embrace cooperative and joyful relationships. This helps in increasing productivity by solving problems amicably. They value the people they work for and with, so they are drawn to those who value relationships and desire to keep those relationships strong.

- *They make the people around them feel comfortable:* They harness tranquility and peaceful coexistence with the people in their circles. They treat others with the respect they deserve regardless of their culture, color, race, status, and academic level. They value whatever engagements other people involve themselves in. Positive people encourage others to pursue their dreams and goals and help others feel supported. This trait promotes congeniality in their relationships.

- *They are a good influence:* Their influence can help you achieve success and life satisfaction as they show by example how to reach your goals. It is common to find people looking up to them because of the kind of life they live and lead. These people will influence you to do those things that add value to your life in terms of empowering you to become productive—making healthy choices such as regular exercise and a nutritious diet; to standing tall in society as a living example to the current and future generations. Whatever they do, they do to the best of their ability so that when they depart from this world, what they have done will live on to influence those whose lives they have touched.

- *They will help you better manage stress:* These personalities tend to offer smiles, laughter, hope, and assurance, which are great treatments for stress. They tend to be good listeners and friends, offering encouragement and support through stressful times. Having cheerleaders like that in our lives can help us return to a place of logical and rational calm after losing our footing. Being around people like that can help us so much when experiencing life's ups and downs.

- *They can help you make better choices because they understand the choices you make today determine how your tomorrow will be:* Positive people will help you to understand life priorities and how to live life in a way that reflects your values. They will, for example, advise you to initiate an exercise routine or encourage you to eat better. But they are also lovers of life, so their diet and exercise will not be bland or boring. They tend to choose delicious, nutritious food to light up the taste buds and find interesting new exercises to add variety to their lives!

- *They keep you away from negativity because they shun it:* They will encourage you to believe in yourself, appreciate failure, and learn a lesson or two from it because, to a positive thinker, failure is not final but an opportunity to begin again. They will also influence you to experience everything you achieve in life, whether success or failure. Because in the end, there is always a lesson to learn from both.

- *Positive people motivate you to follow your dreams and goals:* Dreams are usually inspired by very small ideas, like a tiny seed. However small that seed may be, it will motivate you to stick to your dream. Because out of very small and tiny seeds, enormous trees are produced. They will encourage and support you until you attain your goal. For a seed to grow into a big tree, it must be buried so that it dies, as its death will lead to its germination into a seedling which will then be transplanted, watered, and weeded before it can mature into a giant tree. So is the way to realizing our dreams. Our dreams must undergo those very same stages from the seed stage to mature into full-grown successes!

Expect Good Results, Get Good Results

How often do you sit down and examine your self-expectancy? Self-expectancy is one's expectations of your future ability to carry out or perform a particular assignment or task. Expect your undertakings to be the best they can be. Catch and replace negative thoughts in your brain that aim to convince you that you cannot achieve what you have set out to do. Only allow the best quality thoughts that assure you of great achievements. Train yourself to only listen to productive, encouraging self-talk.

Remember that our own ideas of future performance can influence the outcome of that performance. People with high and positive self-expectancy usually stay focused on being successful in the ventures they get themselves involved in because success is their anticipated outcome. If your expectation is to succeed at a yoga exercise practice, you will have the motivation to keep going with your yoga because your attitude is set to success.

Self-expectancy allows you to get to choose what you envision to happen in the future! This might, however, take some time to practice at first to develop positive self-expectancy. Once you get it down, it becomes part of your daily practice.

A newborn baby does not commence to walk and eat adult food immediately after it is born. It must be breastfed for a couple of months before he or she can be introduced to other important life milestones like eating solid food and the rest of the stages. In yoga exercise, you must begin by taking baby steps to reach small goals, proving to yourself that your larger goals of yoga exercise are indeed attainable in the long run.

It's Never Too Late to Start

Setting your own pace is key to following through on your fitness goals for easy adaptability. No need to say, "it's too late at my advancing age to start a yoga fitness program," because it's never too late to start—even if you have no prior experience.

More importantly, we need to understand that we are not racing to compete and improve. We should always be realistic rather than holding ourselves to unrealistic standards or tight schedules. We should consider setting broader and achievable goals that we can reach over a given period of time. You may want to start by setting a goal to do one yoga pose each day or to feel less pain when lifting things. Whatever goal it is, make sure it is one that is important to you, fits your current state of health and physique, and then you can achieve it—step by step.

Research shows that even those who aren't used to exercising can still experience great results from exercising. One study found that older people who have never exercised regularly have the same ability to build muscle mass as highly trained athletes of a similar age (University of Birmingham, 2019).

What is needed is more specific guidance on how individuals can improve their muscle strength and power, even outside of a gym setting, through activities undertaken in their homes. Such activities as gardening, walking up and down stairs, or lifting a shopping bag can all help improve power if undertaken as part of a regular exercise regimen. This means you can still reap the rewards of exercise even if you have no prior history. And, of course, chair yoga would introduce you to exercise slowly and gently.

The power of positive thinking should not be underestimated because it is a major source of inspiration that helps us attain our goals. So take some time this week to try one of the practices mentioned in this chapter and see how you feel. Whether you are taking 5 minutes in the morning to practice gratitude or catching up with a positive friend, you will be making an important decision for your health. And you will be in the right frame of mind to start your chair yoga journey!

Chapter Three:

Warming Up and Protecting Your Body

Before we dive into the actual practice of chair yoga, it's important to talk about your warm-up and cooldown practices. Warm-ups help prepare your body for stretching, and aerobic activities like walking, running, swimming, and any other physical exercise. Cooldowns, on the other hand, help bring your body back to balance and give a feeling of calm and relaxation after an exercise. In simple terms, they cool down your body after a workout, just as the name suggests.

Preparing your body for exercise makes it easier for your muscles to stretch and gain strength and reduces the risk of injury. Cooling down the body is also a great thing for your muscles. During your workout, your heart pumps blood at a higher rate than normal. It is good to ease your heart rate and blood pressure back to their levels before exercise.

This chapter covers the importance of warming up and cooling down, how to do it correctly, and strategies for protecting the body.

How to Warm Up and Cool Down

Warm-ups prime your cardiovascular system by raising your body temperature and increasing blood flow to your muscles which may also reduce muscle soreness. Other benefits of warming up include:

- Improved oxygen efficiency—Oxygen flow is very important during exercise, and the lack of it can hinder your performance. Your muscles and joints demand more oxygen when performing a physical activity. If they are not supplied with enough oxygen, you start to feel pain, tension, and aches when exercising. This is what we call "Oxygen Debt." Your muscles need oxygen to break down the lactic acid that accumulates there. If there is an insufficient supply of oxygen to your muscles, they overproduce lactic acid, which creates a sensation of fatigue and muscle cramps. Warm-ups encourage fresh oxygen flow in your muscles, aiding in movement performance.

- Body protection—Warming up your body prior to an exercise helps lubricate your joints and release any stiffness from your muscles. This makes your muscles and joints more pliable and able to move through a full range of motion without any struggles.

- Improved blood flow and performance—Warm-up activity helps open up your blood capillaries and increase blood flow to your skeletal muscles. Remember, it is the blood that carries the oxygen that your body requires for lactic acid break down. So, increased blood flow simply means increased oxygen supply to your muscles. This helps reduce fatigue hence being able to withstand longer exercises, which leads to greater performance.

- Faster muscle contraction and relaxation—Warming up your body before performing your actual exercises helps raise your body temperature, improving your nerve transmission and muscle metabolism. This eases the movement in your joints and muscles, thus faster and more efficient performance.

- Mental preparation—Performing a brief warm-up helps prepare your mind making you steady and focused on your body and the exercise. This helps improve your coordination, techniques, skills, and posture during your training sessions. It only takes 5–10 minutes of light activity to warm up your muscles before embarking on an exercise routine. Start by focusing on large muscle groups, like your hamstrings. A well-paced walk for 5–10 minutes, or even light dancing, is enough to prime your body for more in-depth movement. Additionally, cycling slowly on a bike or light jogging in place also does the trick. A good warm-up might induce mild sweating but won't leave you feeling tired before your official exercise. Cooldowns allow you to gradually return to your pre-exercise heart rate and blood pressure. While this is less necessary for yoga practices, which don't raise your heart rate significantly, it can still be an enjoyable way to close out your exercise routine. Cooldowns also give your mind time to settle into the calming experience you get after exercising. This offers your mind and body a sense of peace and relaxation. You can reflect on the experience and anything else you may feel. Other important benefits of cooldowns include:

- Decreased DOMS (Delayed Onset Muscle Soreness)—Although it is normal to experience muscle soreness after an exercise, excess DOMS can be very uncomfortable and painful and may even affect your exercise performance in the future. Taking a few extra minutes to cool down after your workout helps prevent excessive muscle soreness, keeping you more comfortable, relaxed, and ready for your next workout.

- Muscle recovery—After your workout, lactic acid builds up in your muscles, as mentioned before, and this takes time to clear up. Cooling exercises help get rid of the lactic acid build-up from your system. In the process, your muscles relax, allowing energy and body fluids to flow through swiftly without getting "stuck" anywhere to cause cramping. This helps speed up your body's recovery after your workout. Similarly to warming up, to cool down, you'll continue your workout session for about five minutes but at a slower pace. This could mean doing your last few poses more slowly or for shorter periods of time or going for another slow walk afterward.

Body Protection Tips

- Speak to your doctor before participating in yoga if you have any medical conditions or injuries—As much as chair yoga is one the safest and most gentle exercises to take toward achieving your fitness goals, never jump into it without your doctor's advice and getting the green light to do so. Ask your doctor about the exercises you should and should not do. You could even show them the charts in this book to get the okay!

- Go slow initially and avoid overstretching—Any physical activity or exercise is dangerous and may cause serious injuries when done incorrectly. To protect your body, be sure to gently perform all your yoga poses in proper alignment and with complete awareness. Start slowly and work your way up. Do not overdo it. Even if you are flexible enough to go deeper into a certain pose, it doesn't mean you always should.

- Avoid problematic poses—There are several ways to achieve the same objective when it comes to yoga poses. You will find that a couple of poses stretch the same muscle and can be performed by individuals with different activity levels and conditions. Select the level that is appropriate for you. Know your limits, and don't push yourself past your comfort level. You can add any modifications you can think of that feel safe to you. Alternatively, feel free to skip a pose and move on to what you feel is easier for you or best suits your activity level and condition. Avoid end-range positions or taking your stretches to the extreme if you have certain medical conditions.

Pay special attention to the following health problems:

Osteoporosis: Many seniors have joint and bone problems due to muscle and tissue loss. This makes your bones brittle and fragile, which is what we refer to as osteoporosis. To avoid injuries if you have this condition, always ensure that you take your yoga poses and stretches slowly, in a controlled manner, and with complete awareness to lubricate and create space in your joints. In case of a pose that involves twisting, always choose the gentlest variation, and NEVER force yourself into a twisted position using your hands. When performing a pose that involves forward bending from the waist, move from the hip joint without rounding your back, and don't go past 45 degrees. Above all, always avoid impact to the joints and bouncing in any pose.

High or low blood pressure: If you have hypertension or low blood pressure and have to perform a pose that involves moving your head and/or chest upward or downward, be sure to move slowly and with awareness. This allows your body to adapt to the change and avoid dizziness.

Spinal arthritis/bone degeneration and spurs: Always keep your head straight when performing a posture that involves bending backward. Don't let your head fall backward.

- Use props as needed. Don't be afraid of using props like blocks, bolsters, straps, blankets, and other yoga accessories. Using props help provide comfort to your feet and sitz bones, (the bottom part of your pelvis), making it easier to modify your yoga practice to be appropriate for medical needs and activity levels. You can purchase these products at Amazon.com. Enter the prop's name into the search bar and look at the reviews to find the highest quality items.

- Wear loose and comfortable clothing that won't restrict you from moving. Be sure you are warm enough. It is also advisable not to wear shoes and perform all your chair yoga postures barefoot for flexibility and stability reasons. Socks are slippery, while shoes are clunky and inflexible. But if your doctor advises you to wear shoes for a certain condition, please do that!

- Drink plenty of fluids. Keep your body hydrated by drinking enough water before, during, and after your exercises. Inadequate fluid intake leads to dehydration. Dehydration can lead to decreased performance in your exercises because it makes you lose muscular endurance and strength. It could make you feel fatigued and then lazy. The exercise will hence feel more difficult physically and mentally. Dehydration can also trigger muscle cramps, nausea, and headaches. Hydrating your body helps lubricate your joints, spinal cord, and other areas of the body. This also helps with shock absorption, thus protecting your body further.

- Proper breathing while carrying out your exercise. Breathing is key in yoga. We put a lot of emphasis on correct breathing because it helps your body stay connected to your mind and your mind stays focused on the present moment. To reap the most benefits from your yoga practice, ensure being mindful of your breathing techniques as it helps improve coordination and proper body form while performing the poses, keeping the awareness between your body and mind.

- Always do a warm-up before your exercise and cool down after the workout, as described in this chapter. Prepare your body for the activities ahead by warming it up and working toward achieving a complete relaxation of the body and mind through cooldowns. Proper warm-ups and cooldowns will help you release all the tension from your muscles and brain, perform your yoga poses correctly, and reap the benefits of it.

- Listen to your body. If you experience pain or exhaustion, take a break. Yoga exercises and poses are sometimes challenging; however, you shouldn't feel pain when practicing any posture. Pay attention to your body. If you feel any pain while performing a pose, stop immediately. Always work within a pain-free range of motion.

- Above all, enjoyment! After you've learned to take the necessary precautions for your present condition, focus on the enjoyment of exploring your body. Be thankful and happy about what you have, who you are, and what you can achieve.

This book is set up in a way to encourage warming up and cooling down. Chapter 4 showcases some gentle and simple chair yoga poses for you to ease into movement. Chapter 5 takes it up a notch with chair yoga cardio exercises. Chapter 6 is a chair yoga sequence that can be done in under 10 minutes. It starts with a warm-up sequence of chair yoga poses, then goes into a sequence for chair yoga cardio exercises, and ends with a cooldown sequence. When you are pressed for time, you can do the 10-minute sequence, and you will know that you have warming up and cooling down built into the sequence. When you have more time, you could start with all of the Chapter 4 poses and then do all of the exercises in Chapter 5, which does have a cooldown pose at the end. You can also do the suggestions above before and after your chair yoga session, such as a short walk around the block or a gentle and slow bike ride on top of the sequences. Experiment and see what feels right for you. This book was designed in a way to give you snippets of things to do in the time that you have. I have bought and gone through many books with hundreds and hundreds of poses to master, and I have felt really overwhelmed, even with my yoga background. So I did not want my readers to have that experience and kept my book and poses short and sweet!

Now that you know why it is important to warm up and cool down before and after your physical activity, it's time to dive into the practice of chair yoga. Read on to learn about some essential poses, along with tips for making chair yoga a part of your daily routine.

Chapter Four:

15 Simple Poses for Your Daily Routine

In this chapter, you will find simple chair yoga poses with step-by-step instructions on how to execute them and pointers on how to make your yoga practice part of your daily routine. These poses are good for beginners and people looking to slowly and gently improve their flexibility and mobility and gain some balance. They are also great for building body strength gradually. The poses in this chapter are very simple to do. They are a perfect way to begin your chair yoga journey while being kind and gentle to your body.

The instructions may seem like a lot of detail at first. However, within a few repetitions of each, your body will know what to do, and once you get it down, you can just look at the upcoming charts for guidance.

Remember, you don't need any fancy equipment to perform chair yoga. But here are a few optional items that can support your exercise journey!

- Chair: There isn't a specific type of chair that you should use. However, if you can, try to avoid chairs with wheels because they are unstable. Also, a chair without armrests is ideal as the armrests can get in the way. Definitely choose one that is comfortable to sit in and move in. Experiment with the chairs in your home to find the best one. You can also use the end of your couch but make sure the cushion is firm and supportive. If you are shorter and your feet don't reach the ground firmly, look for a shorter chair. You must feel stable and be able to firmly plant your feet on the ground.

- Timer: A timer is handy for timing the poses and exercises. If you have a smartphone, they usually have clock/timer apps that will meet your needs, and you can select a gentle, relaxing bell tone to end each pose and exercise.

- Stopwatch: You may also use a stopwatch instead of a timer. The stopwatch allows you to take the time you need without feeling rushed. Just keep an eye on the time so you don't overextend yourself. Again, look for the clock/timer app on a smartphone, which usually has a stopwatch function.

- Yoga mat: You may place a yoga mat under your chair to help prevent it from sliding on the floor and to cushion your feet to prevent friction. It can also be warmer than the floor on a chilly morning.

Making Yoga a Part of Your Routine

When exercise isn't part of your regular routine, it can sometimes feel difficult to get started or make time in your schedule for it. You might experience some resistance to the thought of getting started or find yourself making excuses for why now "isn't the right time."

Yoga practice can be intimidating, and it is not always easy to get into it or stay consistent with it. You may be willing to try but never find the motivation to do so. So if you are a struggling beginner or someone who has fallen out of your daily exercise routine and wants to get back into it, here are a few things you can do to get and stay hooked on a yoga routine!

- *Use yoga clothes that make you feel good.* Just like in any sporting activity, the assurance of confidence and comfort is key and essential in yoga practice. Wearing loose and comfortable clothes does actually make you more likely to follow through on your workout. If feasible, treat yourself to a few pieces that make you feel like you can breathe and move freely during your practice. Or look in your closet; maybe something you have from your last exercise endeavor will be perfect for your yoga practice!

- *Remind yourself of the benefits.* Yoga is an extraordinary and unique practice compared to other forms of exercise. It has endless unrivaled benefits to your body, soul, and spirit. Whenever you think of skipping yoga, just revisit the benefits discussed in the first chapter of this book.

- *Create your own sequence that feels comfortable and works for you.* Your state of health and flexibility should be your main considerations regarding the choice of yoga sequence you want to practice. There are so many yoga poses with different variations to choose from, and many have benefits for you! Once you have mastered the routines in this book and are confident in your knowledge of chair yoga, then you can experiment with creating your own sequences. Go for the poses you are comfortable doing and best suit your goal.

- *Remember that even 10 minutes is better than nothing.* Start small and do everything you can to practice yoga consistently. Remember, we are talking about making yoga your new habit. Set aside time, even if it is only 10 minutes to practice yoga. Ten minutes is equal to 600 seconds. That can be a very long and productive time in yoga practice. You do not need all the time in the world to do your yoga. Look at your schedule and figure out how much time you can spare to do yoga. A 10-minute session or even just a swift stretch is always better than doing nothing at all! Carve out a small manageable amount of time and make it your sacred "me time." Start small and commit to once or twice a week at first. Then add more sessions as you get into the habit. It takes continuous practice to hone your yoga skills. Start with the easy poses and work your way up. Ideally, three to four times a week. Bonus points for getting into a daily routine! I actually find it easier to start integrating a new habit daily than trying to remember which are my "on" days and which are my "off" days. But do what works for you, do whatever it takes to keep your determination and motivation strong and alive!

- *Remind yourself of your "why."* Successful people are people who can figure out why they do what they do and are able to decide if the things they do are worth doing. For instance, when you start doing yoga, ask yourself what you will be able to achieve when you stick to your yoga practice consistently. Will you be able to spend more time being active with your grandchildren or other children in your life? Or will you be able to travel more and spend more time with your friends? The answers to these tangible questions are very critical to making yoga part of your daily routine. You should write down the reasons and put them strategically somewhere you will be able to see them frequently and regularly.

- *Take a quiet moment to breathe and reflect on the things you're grateful for.* Never underestimate the power of a quick moment spent in silence. Quiet time is a very integral part of life; it affords us the opportunity to reflect on a lot of things that happen in and around our lives. That is why yoga teachers advise their students to find a comfortable place to sit without any distractions and disturbances, close their eyes, take a couple of deep breaths, and allow themselves some ample time to reconnect with themselves. As you focus on your inhale and exhale, you will start to feel relaxed and calm throughout your body. This can create feelings of peace which are so beneficial to the nervous system and all the other systems in the body. If you slip from your chair yoga routine, don't beat yourself up or get frustrated; take some time for deep breathing instead. You may kick off your day with some deep breathing before you get involved in your daily activities or do your deep breathing session as the last thing in the night as your day comes to a close. Ten deep breaths is a great place to start.

- *Practice yoga first thing in the morning.* Taking a couple of deep breaths and stretches when waking up in the morning after enjoying a beautiful night of sleep can make you feel like a million bucks! Starting your day on a high note is awesome because it will keep you going with energy and vitality all day long. Our bodies benefit from yoga and meditation the most in the morning. That is why you are advised to do yoga first thing in the morning. The more time you take to do yoga, the better for your health, but as mentioned before, 10 minutes can do wonders if it is the only time you have.

- *Leave your chair somewhere you'll see it and be reminded to practice.* Remember the adage "out of sight, out of mind." You are likely to forget about your yoga practice if you don't have any visual cues in place. Visual cues are an integral part of habit formation. This is especially true of people who just began practicing yoga or those struggling to keep the habit. If you can, it is best to leave your chair or yoga mat somewhere you can easily see it. This will help remind you that you need to practice your yoga session of the day and help you make it a habit!

- *Create a dedicated space for your practice.* Look for a spacious room or spacious corner of a room that allows stretching and other maneuverings of movements that you will be practicing. Make it a welcoming, enjoyable space for yourself to be in. Maybe decorate it with candles, flowers, or anything else that can give it an inviting feeling for you.

- *Use it as a positive coping mechanism when feeling stressed or overwhelmed.* How are your coping skills when faced with challenges? Do you find it hard to cope with the difficult situations that can appear in life? Try doing a few of the poses in this chapter the next time you feel stressed. Yoga and deep breathing are great remedies for those tough times. Practicing yoga can be like therapy for your body, mind, and soul.

- *Catch yourself when you're making excuses.* You might even consider writing down your most common excuses so you can become more aware of them. At the end of each session, reflect on your accomplishments and the progress you've been making. I find a journal or a log of my daily achievements very helpful in my journey to integrate a new habit.

- *Lay out your yoga clothing the night before and put them on first thing in the morning.* This gets you in the "zone" to do yoga before getting sucked into the other activities of the day. You sort of make a contract with yourself to do yoga that day with this action in the morning.

Before we dive into the actual yoga practice, it's important to know that the emphasis on breathing is what makes yoga so unique and magical when compared to other physical activities. In fact, proper breathing is yoga's main principle; it is one of the most valuable tools for changing the state of your mind. It helps you to stay focused and feel relaxed, maintain heat in the body and good circulation and help you cool down when overheated.

It's important to breathe into your abdomen and not the chest. This is proper diaphragmatic breathing, also called belly breathing. You can practice accessing this breath by putting one hand on your chest and one hand on your belly. You want to feel the belly moving but not the chest. Feel your abdomen expanding out with the in breath like a balloon inflating and moving in with the out breath, like a balloon deflating. You can feel the breath moving through the chest area but avoid having the chest rise and fall with the breath. Use this breath in your poses when you can.

Also, breathe through the nose and not the mouth when you can. Nasal breathing is helpful to the body. Of course, if you have a condition that prevents this, then don't worry about it. But if you can, go for nasal breathing.

One last note: In these yoga poses, I have also added the traditional Indian name when there is one. You might notice that they all end in the word "Asana," which means pose or posture in the Indian language. My yoga teacher explained to me that when you use the Indian name, it's sort of like using the scientific name of a plant species. It's the same—no matter where you go in the world and no matter what language you're speaking. In the English language, we have come up with some cute names that describe the poses, sometimes having to do with an animal, like the dolphin pose and the frog pose. But when you refer to the Indian name, then any yoga practitioner can understand you even if they don't know the English name. So I have the Indian names there to honor the classical, traditional names. But don't let those long Indian words overwhelm you or intimidate you. I just have them there as a reference. You can focus on the English name if that's more comfortable for you!

Now it is time to get your body moving! Let's explore these wonderful poses!

1. Chair Mountain Pose (Chair Tadasana)

As the main principle of yoga practice is proper breathing, the Chair Mountain pose is a great place to start. It helps you practice breathing awareness and calms your body and mind, making you feel more grounded. This pose utilizes your back muscles, shoulders, abs, and the front of your chest, thus helping strengthen and stretch these muscles too.

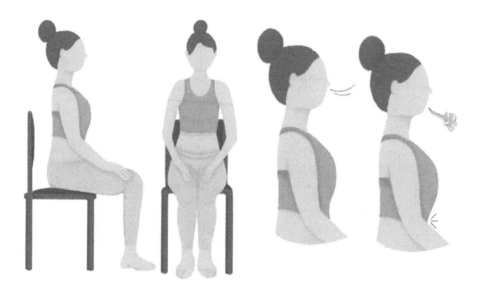

Step-by-Step Instructions:

- Sit up nice and tall in the chair, leaving some space behind you.

- Keep your back straight, spine lengthened, knees bent at a 90-degree angle, and feet flat and firmly planted on the floor hip-width apart.

- Place your hands on your thighs with your palms facing down.

- Keep your shoulders neutral, chest raised, and relax your limbs and face.

- Engage your abdomen slightly and pull your belly button toward your spine and up just a bit.

- Roll your shoulder blades down toward your back and relax your elbows at the sides.

- Now close your eyes and start breathing in and out deeply through your nose. Pay attention to your breathing, and be sure it feels comfortable.

- Continue with this breathing for 10 complete breath cycles. You may also time it for 30 seconds if your mind wanders and you have trouble keeping count.

- Slowly and gently open your eyes and release your hands down by your sides to come out of the pose.

2. Seated Side Stretch

This pose works out your neck, shoulders, arms, and the sides of your torso, which includes your oblique muscles. It is a good exercise if you want to gain joint mobility and flexibility in your arms, shoulders, and upper body. It also helps aid digestion, hence improving metabolism.

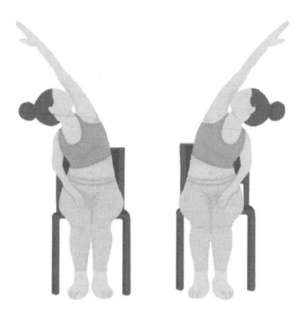

Step-by-Step Instructions

- Sit up nice and tall in the chair toward the chair edge, so your back isn't leaning on it.

- Keep your back straight, spine lengthened, and feet flat and firmly planted on the floor hip-width apart.

- Place your hands on your thighs with palms facing down.

- Keeping both sitz bones firmly planted on the chair seat, bring your right hand and place it palm facedown on your right thigh and reach your left hand up and over to the right facing forward and tilting your torso over slightly to the right.

- Hold here for 3 deep and complete breaths. Listen to your body. Be sure you feel the stretch on the left side of your torso.

- Come back to a neutral position (starting point) by releasing yourself slowly and maintaining an upright spine.

- Switch to the opposite side and hold for 3 deep and complete breaths.

- *Tips:* If you aren't that flexible and need an easier variation, forgo the torso tilt and just raise your arm upward or out to the side. If you are more flexible and need a challenging variation, try placing your hand behind you instead of placing it on your thigh. This adds in more shoulder and chest opening.

3. Chair Cat-Cow Stretch (Chair Marjaryasana Bitilasana)

This is a great stretch to prepare you for other exercises. It benefits and stretches your entire spine, back muscles, shoulders, ab muscles, hips, and pelvic floor muscles. It helps relieve pain from an achy back. It also helps improve posture and balance—and leaves you relaxed and calm. It is a good exercise to begin your chair yoga session with because it helps expand your breath and perk up your entire body.

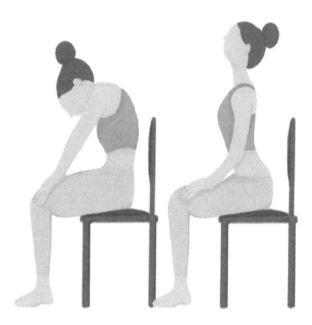

Step-by-Step Instructions:

- Sit up nice and tall at the edge of the chair with your spine lengthened, abdominal muscles engaged, shoulders neutral, and chest raised.

- Plant your feet flat and firmly on the floor hip-width apart with toes pointed straight forward.

- Place your hands just above your knees with palms facing down.

- Carefully and steadily round your chest and spine, scooping your belly inward, curl your tailbone under, then drop your chin toward your chest.

- Arch your spine carefully by bringing your chest outward while sticking your hips out behind you.

- Gently squeeze your shoulder blades together and briefly gaze at the ceiling.

- Repeat 3–10 times depending on your flexibility, training level, and injuries.

Tip: For a more challenging variation, engage the backs of your thighs during the cat pose (when your back is arched). This helps increase the intensity of the stretch.

Caution: Skip this pose if you are still recovering from a serious back injury. However, if you want to try it regardless of your situation, consult your doctor and while executing the pose, please be extremely gentle and be sure to move slowly and with intention. Don't force any pose.

4. Chair Raised Hands Pose (Urdhva Hastasana)

This pose works and benefits your arms, back, shoulders, and even your abdominal muscles. It is a good workout for gaining shoulder joint mobility and flexibility because it helps lubricate the mentioned joints, thus increasing their range of motion. It also helps energize your body and prepare your arms for the day's movements.

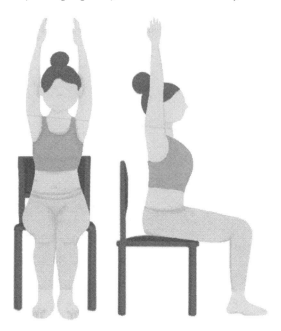

Step-by-Step Instructions:

- Sit up nice and tall in the chair toward the chair edge, so your back isn't tempted to lean on the chair back.

- Keep your back straight, spine lengthened, and feet flat and firmly planted on the floor hip-width apart.

- Place your hands on your thighs with palms facing down.

- Drop your hands to the sides, then raise both arms toward the ceiling.

- Hold here for 1–2 deep breaths, then bring your arms back to your sides in a gentle and controlled manner.

5. Seated Neck Stretch

This exercise stretches your neck and shoulder muscles and can help you regain your mobility and range of motion in the neck muscles and joints. It also helps release stiffness, stress, and tension in these muscles.

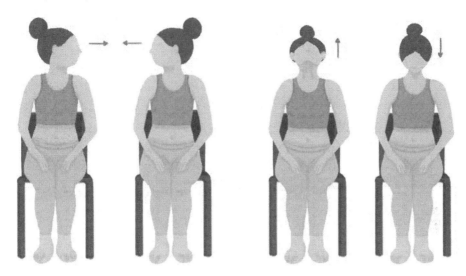

Step-by-Step Instructions:

- Sit up nice and tall toward the edge of the chair with your spine erect and relaxed, feet planted firmly on the floor about hip-width apart.

- Rest your hands on your upper thighs just above your knees with palms facing down and take a deep breath in through your nose, then exhale slowly.

- Next, look side to side, in a slow and gentle movement, 10 times each,

- Then look up and down, in a slow and gentle movement, 10 times each.

6. Seated Shoulder Rolls

The shoulders and neck region seem to be one of the most common areas people store stress. It is important to try to remind yourself to relax your shoulders throughout the day. Shoulder rolls exercise is very helpful for releasing muscle tightness due to stress and tension. It works your neck, shoulders, arms, and upper back. Shoulder rolls are also great for increasing flexibility and mobility in your shoulder joints.

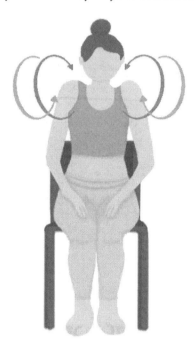

Step-by-Step Instructions:

- Sit up nice and tall in the chair toward the chair edge, so your back isn't tempted to lean on the chair back.

- Keep your back straight, spine lengthened, and feet flat and firmly planted on the floor hip-width apart.

- Place your hands on your thighs with palms facing down.

- Inhale deeply through your nose as you lift both shoulders up toward your ears.

- On an exhale, slowly and gently roll both shoulders back and down in a circular motion.

- Keep rolling your shoulders back and down in a smooth and gentle, continuous motion for 10 rotations or 15 seconds and breathing at a pace that feels good with the movement.

- Then go in the other direction for 10 rotations or 15 seconds.

Tips: If you find it difficult to do the complete rotations, you can raise your shoulders up and down in a shrugging motion instead. You may also start with smaller shoulder circles and work your way toward making fuller circles.

If you have armrests on your chair and your hands are bumping the chair each time you rotate, you can hold them at a 90-degree angle and isolate just by rolling the shoulders back.

7. Chair Pigeon Pose (Chair Eka Pada Rajakapotasana)

Our outer hips, external rotators, and knee joints can really get tight after sitting for hours. Chair pigeon helps strengthen and lubricate your hips and knee joints, hamstrings, glutes, inner thighs, abs, and lower back muscles. This helps relieve tightness and improve flexibility and mobility in the muscles worked. It also helps alleviate pain from sciatica or any irritation of the sciatic nerve.

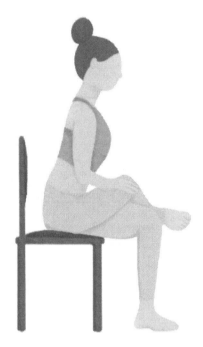

Step-by-Step Instructions:

- Sit up nice and tall toward the edge of the chair with your spine erect and relaxed.

- Plant your feet flat and firmly on the floor hip-width apart, and rest your hands on your lap with palms facing down.

- Bend your right leg and cross it over your left thigh at the right ankle keeping the right knee out to the side.

- Rest your right hand on your shin and the left hand on your right ankle, maintaining a straight back and spine.

- Hold here for 3 deep breaths.

- Then, slowly unwind from the position and bring your torso back to sitting upright.

- Do the other side and hold for 3 breaths

Tips: For an easier variation, just bring your entire right leg and cross it on top of your left thigh. And for a more challenging variation, start in the pose and then slowly and gently tilt your torso forward.

Caution: Skip this pose if you are not flexible enough, or STOP if you experience any degree of pain in your knee and hip joints when trying it.

8. Chair Eagle (Chair Garudasana)

Eagle pose is said to be a good exercise for building focus and concentration. It also works your shoulders, elbows, wrists, upper back, and leg muscles, thus stretching, strengthening, and helping you gain flexibility and mobility in these muscles.

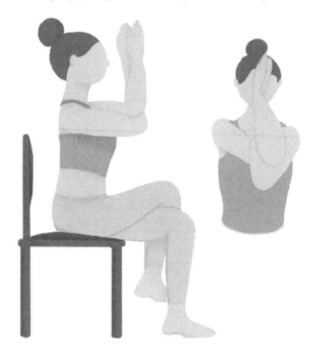

Step-by-Step Instructions:

- Sit up nice and tall toward the edge of the chair with your spine erect and relaxed, feet planted firmly on the floor hip-width apart, and hands rested on your lap.

- Lift your hands to the front of your body and bend your elbows, then cross your upper arms by bringing the left arm on top of the right.

- Wrap your forearms around each other and bring your palms together in front of your face. Be sure that your upper arms are parallel to your thighs.

- Bring your right leg on top of your left thigh such that they are crossed, and try to double-cross your right foot behind the left ankle. (You may rest your right toes toward the floor on the outside of your left foot if your foot can't reach behind your left ankle.)

- Adjust yourself in the chair and be sure that you are sitting upright.

- Draw your abdominals inward and upward to engage your abs, then gaze ahead.

- Hold here for 3 deep breaths.

- Unwrap your arms and legs to release yourself from the cross position and return to sitting upright.

- Do the other side and hold for 3 breaths.

Tips: For an easier variation, simply bring the backs of your hands together instead of bringing your palms together in front of your face. Skip this pose if you are not flexible enough to perform it.

9. Reverse Arm Hold

Reverse arm hold works your chest, shoulders, and arms. It helps open your chest and lubricate your shoulder joints, thus enhancing flexibility and mobility in this area. It also relieves stress and helps people with breathing difficulties.

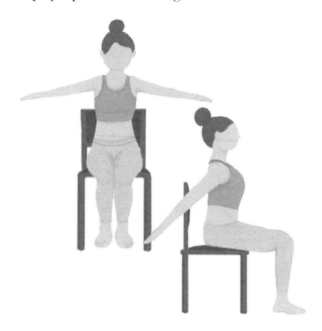

Step-by-Step Instructions:

- Sit up nice and tall toward the edge of the chair, leaving some space behind you.

- Keep your back straight, spine lengthened, knees bent at a 90-degree angle, feet flat and firmly planted on the floor hip-width apart, and your hands rested on your upper thighs with palms facing down.

- Take a deep breath in as you extend your arms straight out to your sides at a low and wide angle.

- On an exhale, roll your shoulders forward and reach your hands behind your back, bending your elbows slightly.

- Slightly bend forward or arch your back to feel the stretch in your shoulders.

- Hold here for 3 complete deep breaths.

- Bring your hands back to the starting point.

10. Chair Spinal Twist (Chair Ardha Matsyendrasana)

This twist helps work your back muscles, neck, and arms. It is good for gaining muscle flexibility and joint mobility in the spine and neck. It also helps relieve tension and stiffness in the surrounding muscles.

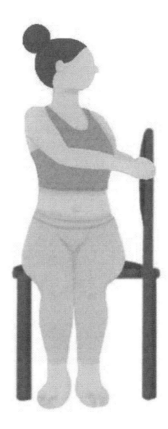

Step-by-Step Instructions:

- Sit up nice and tall sideways in the chair, facing to the left with your spine erect and relaxed.

- Plant your feet flat and firmly on the floor hip-width apart, and rest your hands on your lap with palms facing down.

- Turn to the left, bring both of your hands to the back of the chair and hold the back of the chair as you inhale deeply.

- Exhale as you slowly and gently twist your torso toward the left.

- Hold here for 3 deep breaths.

- Switch sides by moving your legs to the other side and repeat the twist.

- *Tip:* Twisting can be challenging, especially if you are not flexible enough or recovering from a serious injury of the engaged muscles, so always be cautious when trying any twisting pose. Be kind to your body and twist very gently to avoid injuries.

11. Heel Raises

This pose is great if you want to work the opposite sides of your feet and the lower legs. Heel raises recruit your calf muscles and inner thighs, creating a range of motion in the ankle joints. It also helps strengthen your calves and lifts your mood.

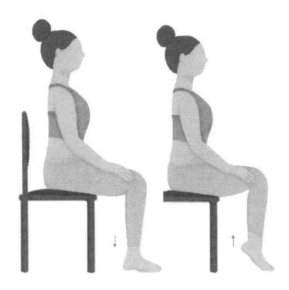

Step-by-Step Instructions:

- Sit up nice and tall toward the edge of the chair with a straight back, spine erect and relaxed.

- Place your hands on your lap, take a deep breath in through your nose and slowly exhale.

- Inhale as you lift both heels, then exhale as you lower them.

- Repeat 3–10 times, depending on your ability.

Tip: You can also alternate your heels by lifting your right heel several times, then your left heel the same number of times, and just play around with the speed.

Seated Tree Pose: Chair Vrksasana

Tree pose is one of the classic yoga poses that is incredible for helping you get grounded and improving your balance, making it easier to go about your daily life. It works and strengthens your arms, core, and legs. Practicing tree pose while sitting in a chair is a great variation for people who are not flexible enough or unable to balance yet. You can still achieve all the benefits of tree pose by practicing while seated in a chair. Here is how you can achieve the three elements of tree pose: balancing, strengthening, and grounding.

12. Seated Tree Pose: Balancing Variation

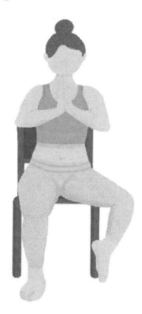

Step-by-Step Instructions:

- Sit up nice and tall toward the edge of the chair with a straight back, spine erect and relaxed.

- Keep your back straight, spine lengthened, and feet flat and firmly planted on the floor hip-width apart.

- Bring the right leg in front of you by extending it slightly forward.

- Bring the left leg out to the side with the heel resting on the front leg of the chair or block and toes planted on the floor.

- Bring your torso slightly forward by hinging at the hips—just a little bit.

- Bring your palms together in front of your chest and gaze forward. Alternatively, you can raise your arms up toward the sky for an extra stretch.

- Hold here for 3 complete deep breaths.

- Then, release yourself from the pose.

- Repeat on the opposite leg.

13. Seated Tree Pose: Grounding Variation

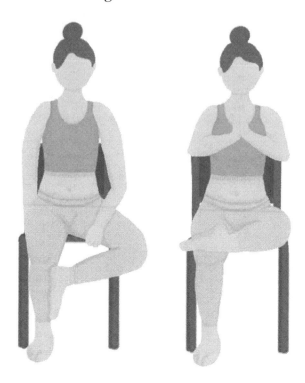

Step-by-Step Instructions:

- Sit up nice and tall toward the edge of the chair with a straight back, spine erect and relaxed.

- Keep your back straight, spine lengthened, and feet flat and firmly planted on the floor hip-width apart.

- Ground your right leg on the floor by pressing your toes into the floor, engaging your thigh.

- Extend your left leg in front of you and bring it onto your right foot with the heel touching the ankle of the right foot.

- If this is intense, you may open your left leg to the side with your foot resting on a block on the floor.

- If you feel flexible enough, you can bring your left foot onto your right thigh to rest just above the knee.

- Now, place one hand on your belly and the other hand on your chest.

- Inhale and exhale deeply while paying attention to your breath and the flow of energy in your engaged muscles. Feel your belly rise and fall but keep your chest still; let the breath go through the chest without much movement but emphasize the belly moving out with the in breath and in with the out breath. Do 3 deep breathing cycles in this manner.

- Unwind yourself and repeat on the opposite leg.

14. Seated Tree Pose: Strengthening Variation

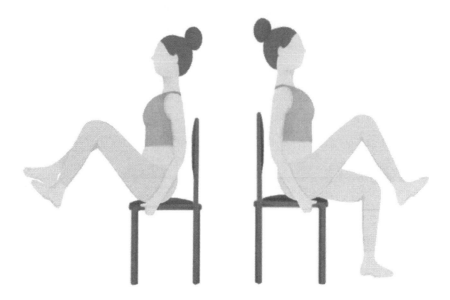

Step-by-Step Instructions:

- Sit up nice and tall toward the edge of the chair with a straight back, spine erect and relaxed.

- Keep your feet flat and firmly planted on the floor hip-width apart.

- Bring your right foot and place it on top of the left foot.

- Extend the left leg in front, keeping its heel planted on the floor with toes pointed upward.

- Hold the sides of the chair and lean slightly backward, engaging your core.

- Lift the left leg a few inches off the floor. Or keep one leg down for support if raising both legs is too much for you.

- Hold here for 1–2 seconds or one deep inhale.

- Exhale as you bring it back to the floor.

- Repeat on the opposite leg.

15. Chair Savasana: Relaxation Pose

This pose will help your body relax and take in all the good results of the poses you have been doing. It calms your mind and helps you cool down and unwind after your yoga session.

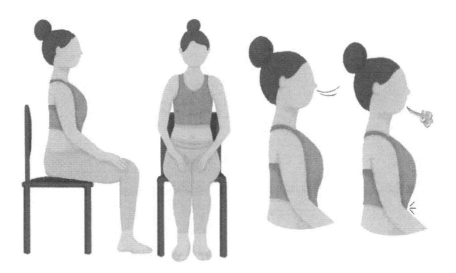

Step-by-Step Instructions:

- Sit up nice and tall in the chair, leaving some space behind you.

- Keep your back straight, feet flat on the floor hip-width apart, and hands resting on your lap with palms facing downward.

- Keep your hands and your entire body relaxed, and close your eyes.

- Breathe naturally through your nose. Focus your attention inward and slow your breathing down.

- Pay attention to relaxing your breathing, allowing any tension in your body to release. Focus on your inhales and exhales.

- You can count your breath and feel your abdomen as it moves in and out on each exhale and inhale.

- Stay in this relaxed position for 10 deep breaths, or set a timer for 30 seconds.

- When you are ready, slowly and gently open your eyes and wiggle your fingers and toes.

- Get up from the chair in a slow and controlled manner to avoid dizziness.

As you practice these moves, you'll get more comfortable with them, and it will become easier to maintain your routine. Don't get discouraged if you aren't motivated at first—putting in the effort will boost your motivation to continue! As they say, every journey begins with a single step or, in this case, a single breath!

The 15 Simple Poses for Your Daily Routine at a Glance

For easy reference during your yoga practice session, here is a chart with images of all the poses described in this chapter at a glance:

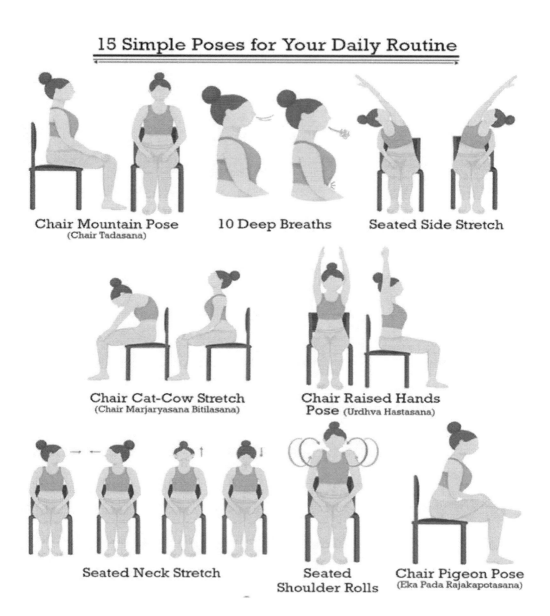

15 Simple Poses for Your Daily Routine

Chair Mountain Pose
(Chair Tadasana)

10 Deep Breaths

Seated Side Stretch

Chair Cat-Cow Stretch
(Chair Marjaryasana Bitilasana)

Chair Raised Hands Pose (Urdhva Hastasana)

Seated Neck Stretch

Seated Shoulder Rolls

Chair Pigeon Pose
(Eka Pada Rajakapotasana)

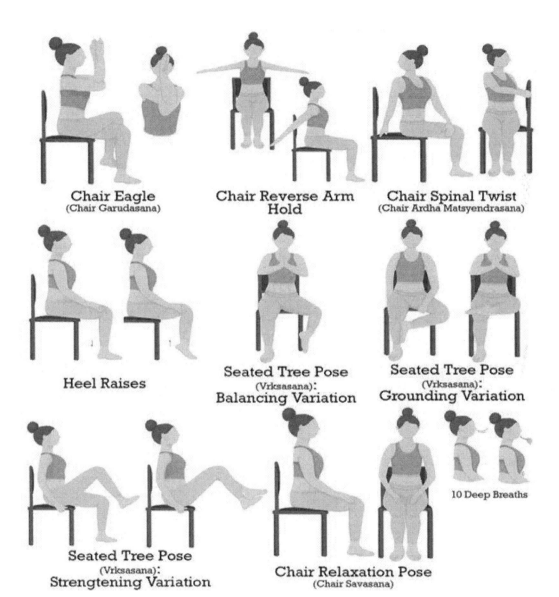

Chair Eagle
(Chair Garudasana)

Chair Reverse Arm
Hold

Chair Spinal Twist
(Chair Ardha Matsyendrasana)

Heel Raises

Seated Tree Pose
(Vrksasana):
Balancing Variation

Seated Tree Pose
(Vrksasana):
Grounding Variation

Seated Tree Pose
(Vrksasana):
Strengtening Variation

Chair Relaxation Pose
(Chair Savasana)

10 Deep Breaths

Can You Help Me Make Someone Else's Golden Years Shine?

"Put knowledge where people trip over it." — *Carla O'Dell*

You might remember from the introduction that my mom is my yoga inspiration. I started teaching her yoga when I was in my late 20s, and nearly 20 years later, she's the most energetic and flexible 80-year-old I know.

My mom wouldn't have come across chair yoga without the knowledge I'd gained throughout my career… and if she had, she wouldn't have known where to look for the guidance she needed. That's why I wrote this book – because I want to share the power of yoga with as many people as possible. It really does have the power to make our golden years shine, and I think that's such an important secret to share.

And this is where I'd like to ask for your help. Just as my mom wouldn't have found the guidance she needed without my help, there are plenty of other people out there who don't know where to find the information they're looking for – or who don't realize how accessible chair yoga really is or how it could transform their lives.

By leaving a review of this book on Amazon, you can help those people leap into their golden years just as energized as my mom.

Just a few sentences telling other readers how this book has helped you and what information you've found here could be the signpost someone is looking for to set them on the right path for amazing flexibility and easy weight loss. And who doesn't want that signpost?

Thank you for helping me on my quest to share the power of yoga with other readers entering their golden years. Our golden years should be just that: shiny and vibrant and full of value. Let's make sure as many people as possible get that benefit.

Chapter Five:

11 Chair Yoga Cardio Exercises for Weight

Loss

If your main goal is to lose excess body fat and achieve lean muscles and a well-toned figure, you may be pondering how chair yoga can help you achieve that with the number of stationary poses involved. The surprising truth of the whole matter is that yoga is one of the more effective regimens for weight loss. Yes, you can use yoga to get rid of stubborn fat buildup—as long as you perform all the poses/exercises involved correctly and stay consistent with your practice. We are also combining yoga poses with chair cardio exercises here to amplify weight loss capability. Later in this chapter, we will discuss the science behind why these poses/exercises and yoga, in general, can help you lose weight.

The exercises in this chapter are inspired by traditional yoga poses, some of which you've previously learned about in this book. They are also inspired by gym-style cardio exercises but performed in a much gentler and more relaxed manner than in a gym setting. Using a chair for support in the comfort of your home and going at your own pace, you can achieve your weight loss goals safely and easily. You can see versions of Chair Hands Raised Pose (Urdhva Hastasana) and Chair Spinal Twist (Ardha Matsyendrasana) from the previous chapter weaved into these poses but with the addition of dynamic movement for added cardio and weight loss capability.

Losing weight is not easy for everyone. In fact, it is easier to gain weight than to lose it. But, this doesn't mean it is impossible to shed off excess body fat. As long as you stay motivated and determined, you can make a huge difference in the way you look and feel.

One thing you need to keep in mind, however, is that exercise alone is not a panacea if you are trying to lose weight. Of course, there are other factors to consider, the major one being your diet. Always remember that just like any other workout routine, you must pair these movements with a healthy diet in order to achieve your weight loss goal. In this chapter, I am going to focus on specific exercises for weight loss that you can easily practice at home. But before we get into that, let's find out how yoga, in general, contributes to weight loss.

Ways in Which Yoga Promotes Weight Loss

Weight change is dictated by energy balance (number of calories consumed versus the number of calories burnt). If you want to lose weight, you will have to burn more calories than you consume. And if you want to gain weight, you need to consume more calories than you burn. To maintain your body weight, you need to consume the same number of calories as those that you burn. So if you are planning to cut your weight, you need to create a calorie deficit. One pound of fat is equivalent to 3,500 calories. This means that the higher the percentage of fat you have, the higher the number of calories you hold in your body. And thus, the higher the number of calories you are required to burn.

Remember, it is much easier to gain weight than to lose it. This means that it is easier to replace calories burnt. You probably have heard the old adage "prevention is better than cure." Yoga has other benefits making it more effective for weight loss than other forms of physical exercise. Yoga can help prevent gaining weight, which is the most important factor.

What does this mean? An individual who burns more calories by performing a high-intensity exercise is more likely to replace them by consuming more calories through mindless eating. But yoga helps prevent this!

To prove this, Alan Kristal, a famous medical researcher and a practicing yogi, conducted a medical study on the effects of yoga on weight loss. In the study, Alan and his colleagues surveyed 15,500 middle-aged men and women about their physical activity (including yoga) and their weight over time. They analyzed the data teasing out other factors that affect weight change, like diet, other forms of exercise, etc.

The results showed that people who practiced yoga regularly lost weight and had fewer chances of gaining weight than people who never practiced yoga. The overweight people who were practicing yoga lost about 5 pounds during that same period, while those who were not practicing yoga gained 14 pounds (Tappenden, 2016).

Kristal and his colleagues discovered that calorie burning doesn't necessarily result in weight loss. You don't necessarily need to burn an adequate number of calories to make a significant difference in your weight. To him, it wasn't clear from the scientific point of view how yoga managed to help people lose weight and keep it low. He noted that yoga has other benefits critical to weight loss that other activities and forms of exercise don't have (Tappenden, 2016). These benefits are discussed below:

Promotes Mindful Eating

Those of us with crazy cravings for certain unhealthy foods know how difficult it is to stop this behavior and how it hurts our chances of losing weight. We already know that healthy foods are good for vibrant living and weight loss. And as much as this knowledge is necessary, just that knowledge alone seems unhelpful in successfully maintaining a healthy eating plan. That's why even those with the most nutritional education may find themselves craving ice cream after 9 p.m. and may not go to bed without having some scoops. Responding to cravings can be like having an out-of-body experience!

One of yoga's special benefits that impacts your eating behavior and weight loss is improved mindfulness of the body and awareness of body sensations. When you do a yoga pose for an extended period of time, you get into a deep connection with your body's feelings. During yoga practice, you are asked to monitor your breath, concentrate on your mind and body, and listen to what they say. By doing so, you are learning and practicing mindfulness.

By practicing mindfulness, you can easily adapt to mindful eating habits. This means you will be able to recognize hunger cues and limit emotional eating, stress eating, and binge eating behaviors that sabotage your weight loss efforts.

With time and practice, you will be able to notice and focus on the foods that make you feel fueled and energized and avoid those with negative effects, including bloating or a lethargic feeling. This can help you stick to a healthy diet or weight loss eating plan.

Several studies have linked yoga practice to improved mindful eating, specifically cutting back on processed junk food and other fast foods and adding more fresh vegetables and other whole foods. One of these studies is a review published in the International Journal of Yoga (Ramos-Jimenez et al., 2015).

Another study published in the Journal of Sports and Exercise Psychology surveyed 159 women who were participating in either regular yoga practice or regular standard exercise. The study found that those who practiced yoga regularly were significantly more likely to have mindful eating patterns than those who did regular standard exercises (Martin et al., 2013).

Yoga is not just about doing physical activity. It is also about listening to your body cues, and this is where it stands out from other physical activities regarding weight loss.

Yoga Can Help Manage Stress That Could Impact Weight Gain

There are several ways in which unmanaged and chronic stress can contribute to weight gain. The breathing techniques and meditation in yoga practice boost your energy and improve your mood, lowering your stress levels.

As discussed earlier, yoga practice also helps increase the secretions of feel-good hormones known as endorphins. These hormones become dominant over the stress-causing hormone cortisol, thus reducing stress.

When you are stressed, your cortisol levels go up. High levels of cortisol hormones lead to increased abdominal fat, a decrease in muscle mass, stress eating, cravings for unhealthy foods, and trouble sleeping. All these can make weight loss very difficult. However, the deep breathing techniques in yoga can help undo and reverse some of these negative effects of stress, which could lead to obesity.

A review from analysis of data from 42 studies published in the Journal of Psychoneuroendocrinology suggested that there is an association between yoga practice and reduced levels of evening cortisol, morning cortisol, heart rate, and cholesterol levels (Pascoe et al., 2017).

Helps Build Muscles

When you hear muscle building, you probably think you must go to the gym and pump iron. Yoga can help you build muscle mass, which in turn helps with weight loss and weight maintenance. By working to keep your body balanced during yoga practice, your muscles get worked out.

Several studies have found yoga to be effective when it comes to muscle building and weight loss. A review of data analyzed from 30 trials with more than 2,000 participants and published in the journal of Preventive Medicine concluded that yoga can reduce body mass index (BMI) in overweight people and reduce waist to hip ratio in healthy adults (Lauche et al., 2016).

Another study found that even practicing slower, restorative yoga, like chair yoga, improves fasting glucose levels in overweight people. This is a sign of good metabolic health (Kanaya et al., 2014).

Stimulate the Crucial Force of the Liver

Your liver is one of the most important organs in your body. It performs so many functions. In fact, it is the largest internal organ in your body and extremely important. It is a powerful cleanser and detoxifier of your body. It processes all kinds of fats and purifies your blood. It also secretes bile juice, which plays an important role in digestion.

If your liver is strong and healthy, it means you will be able to eliminate bad fats from your body and make good fats work better for you. Your liver also stores glucose and stimulates coenzyme Q10 production; these two important elements power your muscles, giving you the much-needed energy to digest food and perform other bodily functions. Practicing yoga helps strengthen your liver's vital force in many ways that bring about optimal functionality. Many verified studies show that yoga stimulates the liver and keeps it healthy.

So you see, yoga is an effective and important part of your daily workout routine; it's crucial if you are unable to do other exercises. The mindfulness and stress reduction benefits of yoga practice enhance better eating habits, increased self-awareness, and improved sleep, which helps with weight loss and maintaining a healthy body shape. Always remember that exercise is just a fraction of the equation, and nutrition and mental well-being are the other parts of the equation. No matter the type of workout you perform, be sure to pair it with a good diet and also be sure to manage your stress levels. We have touched on mental well-being in previous chapters, and we will discuss nutrition more in depth in the last chapter.

Walking daily can also help with weight loss!

Besides yoga practice, regular walking can also help with weight loss. Research indicates that a few 30-minute walks every week can help cut down a considerable amount of body fat and improve your overall cardio fitness (Osei-Tutu & Campagna 2005). Another study published in the American Journal of Sports Medicine showed that a group of women walking daily for six months lost an average of 17 pounds (Gwinup, 1987).

So, simply putting one foot in front of the other can remarkably affect your weight loss goal. You don't have to walk for hours and cover miles. If you are just starting, a 20-minute, steady-paced walk a few days a week or walking for 5 minutes several times a day can do you wonders. As you get used to it, become more flexible and gain more endurance, you will want to raise your routine to a higher level. Here are some tips to motivate you and help you get great results from your walking exercise:

- **Add in some incline**

    - Although regular walking on a flat surface can help you burn calories, adding in some incline can make it more challenging and beneficial. Your body is capable of storing energy in tendons, joints, muscles, and other tissues during walking and uses that energy to propel you forward. This allows you to walk great distances with minimal effort. With this information in mind, you may want to make your walking exercise a bit more challenging. Try to add in some incline by walking up a hill, climbing stairs, or anything that can add some difficulty. This gives your body new stimuli to adapt to. If you are capable of walking on an incline without pain, this can help you achieve your weight loss goals.

- **Get a dog**

    - Becoming a pup parent can be the best motivation for walking. Dogs are great companions and bring joy to your life, and most dogs need a whole lot of movement. Owning a dog will help you exercise more because you will need to take it out for walks.

    - The most recent survey conducted on over 2,000 dog owners found that the average dog owner covers 1,000 miles with their dog every year. This means that by the time your pup is five years old, you will have walked 3,000 miles with him (Renner, 2022). Multiply this by the number of calories an average person burns per mile, and you will have burned 300,000 calories in that time!

    - Another study that targeted older adults specifically analyzed over 3,000 seniors. They found that dog parents were consistently more active than those who didn't own a dog. Those without dogs were more likely to spend their entire day sitting (Wu et al., 2017).

- **Increase the intensity with intervals**

  - If you want to add some challenge to your walking exercise but don't want to climb up a hill or stairs, consider adding in some short intervals of high intensity. For example, walk on your usual flat ground for 10 minutes and then walk at a brisker speed for one minute. Keep alternating between walking at a normal pace and then at an increased speed. This helps increase your heart rate and burn more calories.

  - In fact, research published in the Cell Metabolism Journal found that older adults were able to reverse muscle loss on the cellular level through interval training (walking, cycling) (Robinson et al., 2017). Interval walking can help you burn fat and maintain lean muscle mass.

- **Walk with purpose**

  - If you want to walk longer, have a purpose, for your, walk in mind. Don't just walk aimlessly. A study conducted on over 120,000 people found that walking for a utilitarian purpose has a significant effect on health. It makes you feel healthier, and you'll find it easier to keep going (Pae & Akar, 2020). Commuting to work is a great purpose for walking. But since most seniors are retired or don't work, walking to the grocery store or visiting friends at a scheduled time could do them good.

- **Bring your headphones with you**

  - Music can be a great motivating factor for your exercise. Several studies have found that music can help you overcome fatigue, enable you to exercise longer, and help you enjoy exercise more. One study found that listening to self-selected motivational or upbeat music can help improve endurance and performance even when mentally fatigued (Lam et al., 2021). Since the study focused on running, which is more strenuous than walking, there is no doubt that music can help with walking performance and consistency. So next time you feel tired and ready to skip a walk, try popping in some headphones, throw in your favorite tunes, and hit the road!

Chair Yoga Cardio Exercises for Weight Loss

These poses are a little bit advanced, more active, and bring some cardio in for weight loss. Be sure to always go at your own pace and don't do anything that causes pain! Be very, very careful! If there is any pain, STOP! Always check with your doctor before starting any new exercises. Also, remember that successful weight loss comes from consistent workouts, a healthy diet, managing stress levels, and keeping your body moving. All this together can lead to increased metabolism and burning of fat.

Don't push yourself too hard, and enjoy the process. If anything is painful, go back to the gentler first routine until you have built up some flexibility and strength. That routine should also build up upper body tone. When you return to this routine, go slow, and you can always pick and choose the ones that feel easy and safe for you and skip the ones that don't feel right for your body!

1. Press and Open

This workout is great if you want to lose some stubborn fat buildup on your thighs and improve strength in your arms and legs. It also helps lubricate your shoulder joints, improving flexibility and mobility of the joints and building some muscles on your thighs and hands. This exercise works out your shoulders, hamstrings, quads, triceps, and biceps.

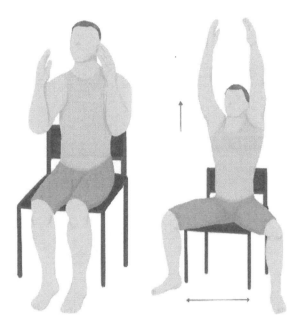

Step-by-Step Instructions:

- Sit up in the chair, nice and tall. Move slightly forward in the chair to leave some space behind you to ensure you are not leaning on the back of the chair.

- Keep your back straight, knees bent and together, feet pointed with toes lightly touching the floor, your arms open in front of you shoulder-width apart, elbows bent at a 90-degree angle, and palms facing each other.

- Lift your legs 1–2 inches above the ground and open them out, flexing your feet and extending them to the sides as you raise your arms up above your head at the same pace.

- Bring your hands back and your legs together at the same pace.

- Repeat for 30 seconds or 15 seconds for beginners or those with injuries.

2. Seated Side Crunch (Left Side)

Side crunches are the best exercises if you want to lose belly fat and build a strong core without putting any strain on your neck, back, or your knees. It helps activate and tone your transverse abdominis and internal and external oblique muscles. If you have never tried a seated ab workout before, give this one a try and see how you like it.

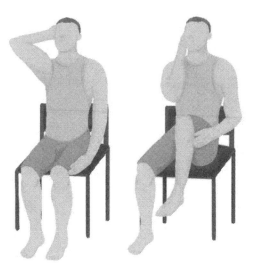

Step-by-Step Instructions:

- Sit up in the chair, nice and tall. Move slightly forward in the chair to leave some space behind you to ensure you are not leaning on the back of the chair.

- Keep your back straight, feet firmly planted and flat on the floor hip-width apart.

- Place your right hand over your right ear and use your left hand to hold the space under your left thigh at the knee joint. Or place your hand behind you and hold the chair for support if needed.

- Raise your left knee toward the right elbow. Be sure to maintain a straight back and engage your abdominal muscles.

- Return your knee back to the starting position.

- Perform 10 reps or repeat for 30 seconds or 15 seconds for beginners or those with injuries.

3. Seated Side Crunch (Right Side)

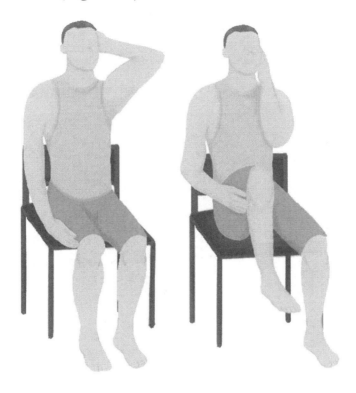

Step-by-Step Instructions:

- Sit up in the chair, nice and tall. Move slightly forward in the chair to leave some space behind you to ensure you are not leaning on the back of the chair.

- Keep your back straight, feet firmly planted and flat on the floor hip-width apart.

- Place your left hand over your left ear and use your right hand to hold the space under your right thigh at the knee joint. Or place your hand behind you and hold the chair for support if needed.

- Raise your right knee toward the left elbow. Be sure to maintain a straight back and engage your abdominal muscles.

- Return your knee back to the starting position.

- Perform 10 reps or repeat for 30 seconds or 15 seconds for beginners or those with injuries.

4. Sitting Jacks

This exercise is perfect for you if you want to get a cardio boost during your chair yoga session. It gives you a little workout without putting pressure on or impacting your joints. It also helps lubricate your shoulder joints and knees, making them more flexible and mobile.

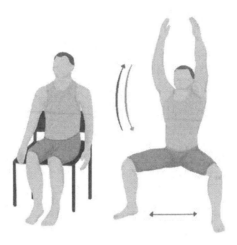

Step-by-Step Instructions:

- Sit up in the chair, nice and tall. Move slightly forward in the chair to leave some space behind you to ensure you are not leaning on the back of the chair.

- Keep your back straight, knees bent and together, feet pointed with toes lightly touching the floor, your arms by your sides with slightly bent elbows and palms facing your legs.

- Quickly but gently open your legs out, flexing your feet and extending them to the sides, raising your arms up above your head at the same pace.

- Bring your hands back to the sides and your legs together at the same pace.

- Repeat for 30 seconds or 15 seconds for beginners or those with injuries.

Tip: If you are a beginner, you can initially start it slow and then eventually increase the speed to a more dynamic, fast-paced range of motion.

5. Step Out and Press

This workout helps stretch and strengthen your leg and arm muscles. It engages several muscle groups in your lower and upper body, including ankles, calves, toes, quads, hamstrings, biceps, triceps, shoulders, and shins. It also helps relieve stiffness and pain in those areas.

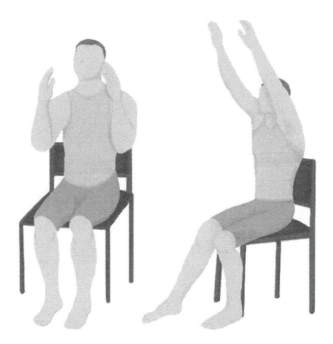

Step-by-Step Instructions:

- Sit up in the chair, nice and tall. Move slightly forward in the chair to leave some space behind you to ensure you are not leaning on the back of the chair.

- Keep your back straight, knees bent, feet pointed hip-width apart with toes lightly touching the floor, your arms open by your sides with elbows bent at a 90-degree angle, and palms facing each other.

- Lift your right foot a few inches off the floor and extend your leg in front of you, pointing your toes forward and flexing your foot as you raise both your arms above your head at the same time.

- Bring your hands and leg back and repeat on the other leg.

- Keep doing it for 30 seconds, then rest. Or 15 seconds for beginners or those with injuries.

6. Seated Chest Claps

This workout helps strengthen your hand and chest muscles. It also helps lubricate your shoulder joints, hence improving flexibility and mobility of the joint.

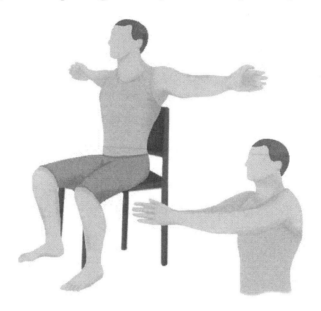

Step-by-Step Instructions:

- Sit up in the chair, nice and tall. Move slightly forward in the chair to leave some space behind you to ensure you are not leaning on the back of the chair.

- Keep your back straight, knees bent, feet flat and firmly planted on the floor hip-width apart with your arms by your sides.

- Extend your arms straight out to the sides at chest level with palms facing forward.

- Bring your palms together as if you are clapping, and lightly touch your hands together.

- Pull your palms away from each other and take your hands back to the starting position. Be gentle with your back, don't squeeze your shoulder blades all the way together with each movement, let the shoulder blades be relaxed as you move.

- Repeat for 30 seconds or 15 seconds for beginners or those with injuries.

7. Lateral Raises Step Outs

This exercise works out your back, hips, shoulders, hands, biceps, triceps, and ab muscles (obliques, transverse abdominis, etc.). It helps gain strength, flexibility, and mobility in the muscles engaged. It also helps relieve anxiety, stress, and tension.

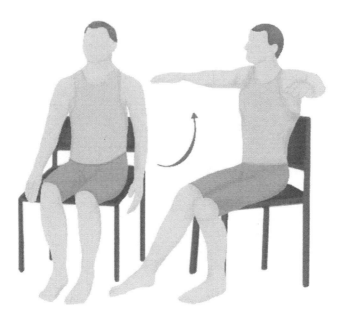

Step-by-Step Instructions:

- Sit up in the chair, nice and tall. Move slightly forward in the chair to leave some space behind you to ensure you are not leaning on the back of the chair.

- Keep your back straight, knees bent and together, feet flat and firmly planted on the floor, and your arms by your sides with a slight bend in your elbows and palms facing your legs.

- Lift your right foot a few inches off the floor and extend your leg in front of you, pointing your toes forward and flexing your foot as you raise both arms at the same time until your elbows are at shoulder height or slightly below your shoulders such that your palms are facing the floor.

- Bring your hands and leg back and repeat on the other leg.

- Keep doing it for 30 seconds, then rest. Or 15 seconds for beginners or those with injuries.

8. Chair Marching

This exercise is perfect for you if you struggle with walking and climbing up and down the stairs or if you sit for prolonged periods. It works your hip flexors, strengthening them and making them more flexible. It gets your legs moving, boosting your metabolism.

In yoga practice, we concentrate on large muscle groups. And this exercise gets your lower half large muscles warmed up, including your core, external rotators, quads, and inner thighs.

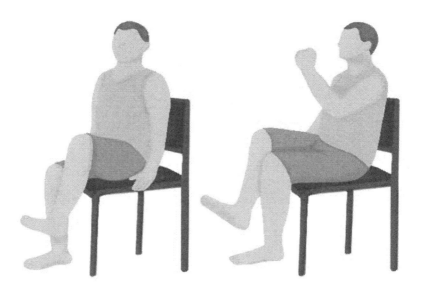

Step-by-Step Instructions:

- Sit up in the chair, nice and tall. Move slightly forward in the chair to leave some space behind you to ensure you are not leaning on the back of the chair.

- Keep your back straight, feet flat on the floor hip-width apart, with your arms by your sides.

- Alternate lifting your legs up and down while pumping your arms as if you are marching up and down the stairs.

- Keep doing it for 30 seconds, then rest. Or 15 seconds for beginners or those with injuries.

- Alternatively, you can omit the arms and only march the legs if doing both the arms and the legs feels like too much.

9. Seated Torso Twist

Twists can be very beneficial for your spine and entire torso. They also help us create flexibility in our neck muscles. Twists are also very helpful if you feel lethargic and need to refresh or have a sluggish digestive system or metabolism. The twisting motion of seated torso twists helps lubricate the spine and open up your back, shoulders, and hips, relieving any tension and stiffness that may be caused by stress, trauma, or injury. They also help you gain a new perspective and increase the range of motion in the intervertebral discs, thus enhancing flexibility and mobility in these muscles. In general, seated torso twists work your neck, spine, back, hips, and oblique muscles.

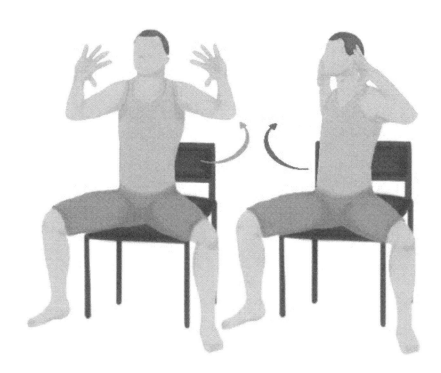

Step-by-Step Instructions:

- Sit up in the chair, nice and tall. Move slightly forward in the chair to leave some space behind you to ensure you are not leaning on the back of the chair.

- Keep your back straight, feet flat on the floor hip-width apart, and hands on your lap with palms facing down.

- Raise your arms out to the sides, bend your elbows, and spread the fingers wide next to your head.

- Push your elbows back, engage your abs, and twist to the left, then back to the center, then to the right.

- Continue this motion for 30 seconds, then rest. Or 15 seconds for beginners or those with injuries.

10. Seated Arm Swings

Arm swings are an amazing dynamic stretching exercise that works out your upper body muscles. They help stretch, strengthen, and warm up your shoulders, arms, chest, and upper back. They also give you a great cardio boost that helps burn some calories and helps lubricate and increase flexibility and mobility in your shoulder joints.

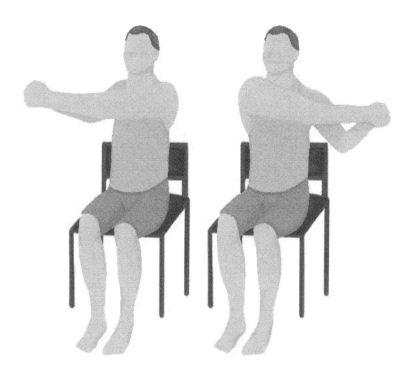

Step-by-Step Instructions:

- Sit up in the chair, nice and tall. Move slightly forward in the chair to leave some space behind you to ensure you are not leaning on the back of the chair.

- Keep your back straight, feet flat and firmly planted on the floor hip-width apart, with your palms on your thighs and shoulders relaxed.

- Extend your arms straight in front of you, bring your palms together, interlocking your fingers or simply putting one palm on top of the other and engage your core.

- Now, start swinging your arms slowly from side to side. Only go as far as is comfortable in the movement.

- Keep doing it for 30 seconds, then rest. Or 15 seconds for beginners or those with injuries.

11. Chair Savasana: Relaxation Pose

This is a perfect pose to help you relax your body, calm down your spirit and unwind your mind after your exercises. Chair Savasana relaxation pose makes you feel good and gives your body time to start integrating the results of your exercises.

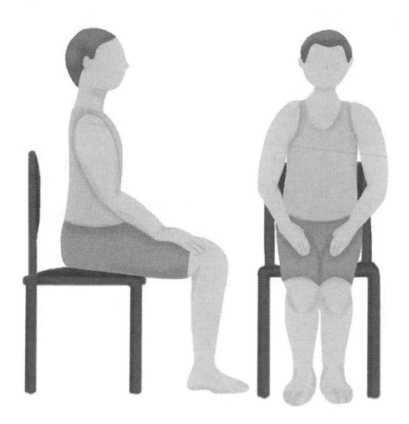

Step-by-Step Instructions:

- Sit up nice and tall in the chair, leaving some space behind you.

- Keep your back straight, feet flat on the floor hip-width apart, and hands resting on your lap with palms facing downward.

- Keep your hands and your entire body relaxed, and close your eyes.

- Breathe naturally through your nose. Focus your attention inward and slow your breathing down.

- Pay attention to relaxing your breathing, allowing any tension in your body to release. Focus on your inhales and exhales.

- You can count your breath and feel your abdomen as it moves in and out on each exhale and inhale.

- Stay in this relaxed position for 10 deep breaths, or set a timer for 30 seconds.

- When you are ready, slowly and gently open your eyes and wiggle your fingers and toes.

- Get up from the chair in a slow and controlled manner to avoid dizziness.

The 11 Yoga Exercises for Weight Loss at a Glance

For easy reference during your yoga practice session, here is a chart with images of all the poses described in this chapter at a glance:

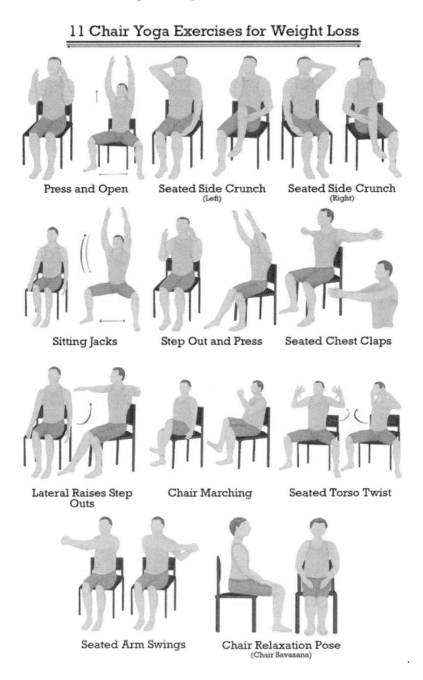

11 Chair Yoga Exercises for Weight Loss

Press and Open   Seated Side Crunch (Left)   Seated Side Crunch (Right)

Sitting Jacks   Step Out and Press   Seated Chest Claps

Lateral Raises Step Outs   Chair Marching   Seated Torso Twist

Seated Arm Swings   Chair Relaxation Pose (Chair Savasana)

Now you have many tricks up your sleeve to lose excess body fat. Next, we'll look at a simple routine you can practice in under 10 minutes, fitting it into any time of your day

Chapter Six:

Chair Yoga in Under 10 Minutes

Having a routine for your yoga sessions is the most effective way to put everything you've learned concerning yoga into practice and benefit from the information presented in this book. In this chapter, I'll share a yoga routine incorporating a full quick workout. I will start with some of the gentler yoga poses to warm up, then go into the chair cardio exercises, and end with more gentle yoga poses to cool down. This may take you longer than 10 minutes the first few times you do this, but soon you won't need the instructions anymore, and then you can breeze through it quickly. After that, you will be able to execute a very swift routine at any time convenient for you, just using the chart at the end or just from memory.

You can use the knowledge you've gained from this book to create your own program. But I recommend you try this one for a few weeks before coming up with your own, especially if you are a beginner. The reason for this is that you need to understand how your body responds to a yoga practice before creating your own routine. I have tried and tested the routines detailed in this book, and I believe it to be a great program for everyone, especially newcomers. They build into each other slowly to help you progress correctly and safely. Once you feel confident about your body's ability to do these poses and exercises properly, then go ahead and start experimenting with different routines. Without further ado, let's get into it!

Warm-Up Sequence

This sequence consists of poses that will help lubricate your joints, warm up your muscles, release any stiffness, and generally prepare you physically and mentally for the rest of the movements. They are a gentle way to get your body moving before you start the other sequences.

1. Chair Mountain Pose (Chair Tadasana), 10 Deep Breaths

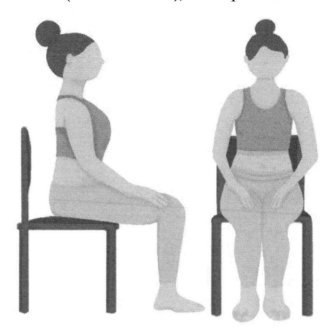

Step-by-Step Instructions:

- Sit up nice and tall in the chair, leaving some space behind you.

- Keep your back straight, spine lengthened, knees bent at a 90-degree angle, and feet flat and firmly planted on the floor hip-width apart.

- Place your hands on your thighs with your palms facing down.

- Keep your shoulders neutral, chest raised, and relax your limbs and face.

- Engage your abdomen slightly and pull your belly button toward your spine and up just a bit.

- Roll your shoulder blades down toward your back and relax your elbows at the sides.

- Now close your eyes and start breathing in and out deeply through your nose. Pay attention to your breathing and ensure it feels comfortable.

- Continue with this breathing for 10 complete deep breath cycles.

- Slowly and gently open your eyes and release your hands down by your sides to come out of the pose.

2. Chair Raised Hands Pose (Chair Urdhva Hastasana), 10 Deep Breaths

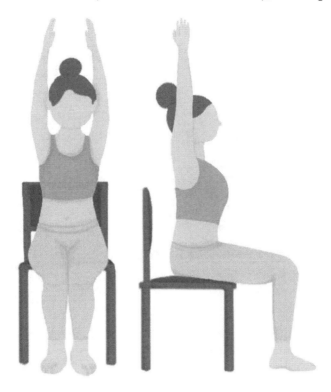

Step-by-Step Instructions:

- Sit up nice and tall in the chair toward the chair edge, so your back isn't tempted to lean on the chair back.

- Keep your back straight, spine lengthened, and feet flat and firmly planted on the floor hip-width apart.

- Place your hands on your thighs with palms facing down.

- Drop your hands to the sides, then inhale as you raise both arms toward the ceiling.

- Hold here for one or two seconds, then exhale as you bring your arms back to your sides in a gentle and controlled manner.

- Repeat 10 times, breathing deeply each time.

3. Chair Cat-Cow Stretch (Chair Marjaryasana Bitilasana), 10 Times in Each Direction

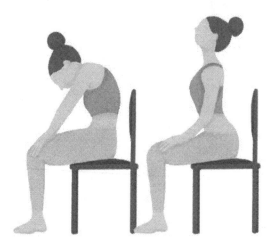

Step-by-Step Instructions:

- Sit up nice and tall at the edge of the chair with the spine lengthened, abdominal muscles engaged, shoulders neutral, and chest raised.

- Plant your feet flat and firmly on the floor hip-width apart, with toes pointed straight forward.

- Place your hands just above your knees with palms facing down.

- Carefully and steadily round your chest and spine, scooping your belly inward, curl your tailbone under, then drop your chin toward your chest.

- Arch your spine carefully by bringing your chest upward while sticking your hips out behind you.

- Gently squeeze your shoulder blades together and briefly gaze at the ceiling.

- Repeat 10 times in each direction.

Tip: For a more challenging variation, engage the backs of your thighs during the cat pose (when your back is arched). This helps increase the intensity of the stretch.

Caution: Skip this pose if you are still recovering from a serious back injury. However, if you want to try it regardless of your situation, consult your doctor and while executing the pose, please be extremely gentle and be sure to move slowly and with intention. Don't force any pose.

4. Seated Neck Stretch, 10 Times in Each Direction

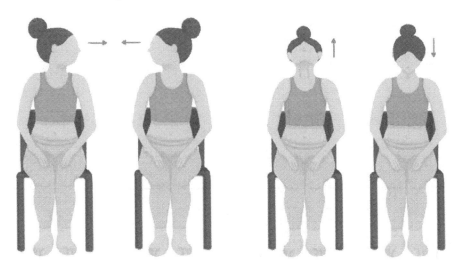

Step-by-Step Instructions:

- Sit up nice and tall toward the edge of the chair with your spine erect and relaxed, with feet planted firmly on the floor about hip-width apart.

- Rest your hands on your upper thighs just above your knees with palms facing down and take a deep breath in through your nose, then exhale slowly.

- Next, look side to side, in a slow and gentle movement, 10 times each,

- Then look up and down, in a slow and gentle movement, 10 times each.

5. Seated Shoulder Rolls, 10 Times in Each Direction

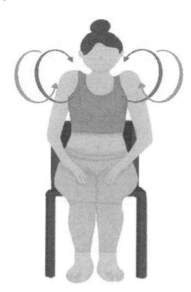

Step-by-Step Instructions:

- Sit up nice and tall in a chair toward the chair edge, so you aren't tempted to lean on the chair back.

- Keep your back straight, spine lengthened, and feet flat and firmly planted on the floor hip-width apart.

- Place your hands on your thighs with palms facing down.

- Inhale deeply through your nose as you lift both shoulders up toward your ears.

- On an exhale, slowly and gently roll both shoulders back and down in a circular motion.

- Keep rolling your shoulders back and down in a smooth and gentle, continuous motion for 10 rotations or 15 seconds and breathing at a pace that feels good with the movement.

- Then go in the other direction for 10 rotations.

If you have armrests on your chair and your hands are bumping the chair each time you rotate, you can hold them at a 90-degree angle and isolate just by rolling the shoulders back.

The Sequence for Cardio

The chair cardio sequence is a short routine for each exercise, so it gives you a snippet of activity to start the day with. Just a little segment of getting the heart rate going and the breath pumping.

1. Seated Chest Claps, 10 of Them

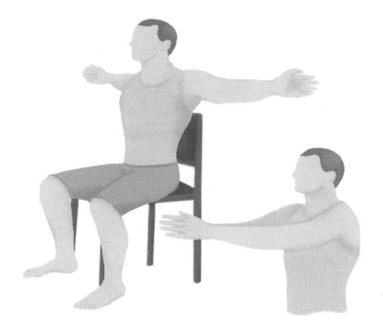

Step-by-Step Instructions:

- Sit up in the chair, nice and tall. Move slightly forward in the chair to leave some space behind you to ensure you are not leaning on the back of the chair.

- Keep your back straight, knees bent, feet flat and firmly planted on the floor hip-width apart, with your arms by your sides.

- Extend your arms straight out to the sides at chest level with palms facing forward.

- Bring your palms together as if you are clapping, and lightly touch your hands together.

- Pull your palms away from each other and take your hands back to the starting position. Be gentle with your back, don't squeeze your shoulder blades all the way together with each movement, let the shoulder blades be relaxed as you move.

- Repeat 10 times.

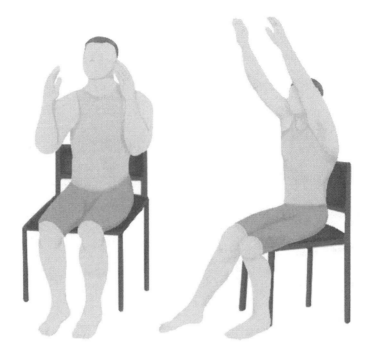

Step-by-Step Instructions:

- Sit up in the chair, nice and tall. Move slightly forward in the chair to leave some space behind you to ensure you are not leaning on the back of the chair.

- Keep your back straight, knees bent, feet pointed hip-width apart with toes lightly touching the floor, your arms open to the sides with elbows bent at a 90-degree angle, and palms facing each other.

- Lift your right foot a few inches off the floor and extend your leg in front of you, pointing your toes forward and flexing your foot as you raise both your arms above your head at the same time.

- Bring your hands and leg back and repeat on the other leg.

- Perform 10 reps on each leg, alternating your legs.

3. Side Crunch to the Left, 10 of Them

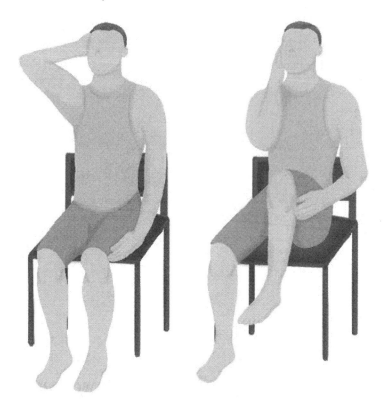

Step-by-Step Instructions:

- Sit up in the chair, nice and tall. Move slightly forward in the chair to leave some space behind you to ensure you are not leaning on the back of the chair.

- Keep your back straight, feet firmly planted and flat on the floor hip-width apart.

- Place your right hand over your right ear and use your left hand to hold the space under your left thigh at the knee joint. Or place your hand behind you and hold the chair for support if needed.

- Raise your left knee toward the right elbow. Be sure to maintain a straight back and engage your abdominal muscles.

- Return your knee back to the starting position.

- Perform 10 reps or repeat for 30 seconds or 15 seconds for beginners or those with injuries.

4. Side Crunch to the Right, 10 of Them

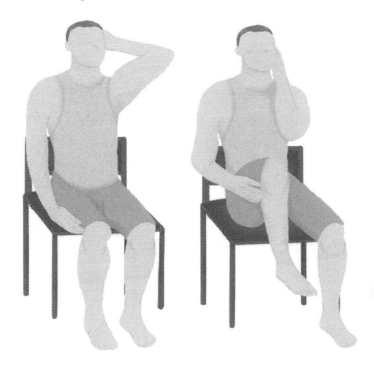

Step-by-Step Instructions:

- Sit up in the chair, nice and tall. Move slightly forward in the chair to leave some space behind you to ensure you are not leaning on the back of the chair.

- Keep your back straight, feet firmly planted and flat on the floor hip-width apart.

- Place your left hand over your left ear and use your right hand to hold the space under your right thigh at the knee joint. Or place your hand behind you and hold the chair for support if needed.

- Raise your right knee toward the left elbow. Be sure to maintain a straight back and engage your abdominal muscles.

- Return your knee back to starting position.

- Perform 10 reps or repeat for 30 seconds or 15 seconds for beginners or those with injuries.

5. Lateral Raise Step Outs, 10 of Them

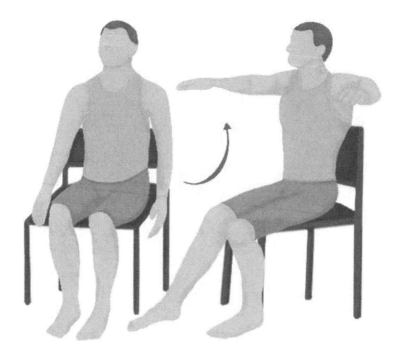

Step-by-Step Instructions:

- Sit up in the chair, nice and tall. Move slightly forward in the chair to leave some space behind you to ensure you are not leaning on the back of the chair.

- Keep your back straight, knees bent and together, feet flat and firmly planted on the floor, and your arms by your sides with a slight bend in your elbows and palms facing your legs.

- Lift your right foot a few inches off the floor and extend your leg in front of you, pointing your toes forward and flexing your foot as you raise both arms at the same time until your elbows are at shoulder height or slightly below your shoulders such that your palms are facing the floor.

- Bring your hands and legs back and repeat on your other leg.

- Perform 10 reps on each leg or repeat for 30 seconds or 15 seconds for beginners or those with injuries.

Cooldown Sequence

This sequence consists of poses that have a more meditative and calming quality in them. You will be asked to hold some of the poses for longer than you have for the previous poses. This will give you a chance to focus your attention inward, enabling you to feel calm and relaxed.

1. Seated Shoulder Rolls, 10 in Each Direction

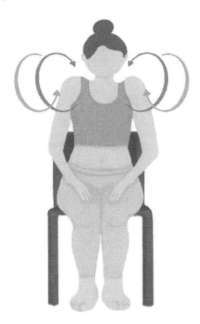

Step-by-Step Instructions:

- Sit up nice and tall in a chair, toward the edge so that you aren't tempted to lean on the chair back.

- Keep your back straight, spine lengthened, and feet flat and firmly planted on the floor hip-width apart.

- Place your hands on your thighs with palms facing down.

- Inhale deeply through your nose as you lift both shoulders up toward your ears.

- On an exhale, slowly and gently roll both shoulders back and down in a circular motion.

- Keep rolling your shoulders back and down in a smooth and gentle, continuous motion for 10 rotations or 15 seconds and breathing at a pace that feels good with the movement.

- Then go in the other direction for 10 rotations.

- If you have armrests on your chair and your hands are bumping the chair each time you rotate, you can hold them at a 90-degree angle and isolate just rolling the shoulders back.

2. Chair Raised Hands Pose (Chair Urdhva Hastasana), 10 Deep Breaths

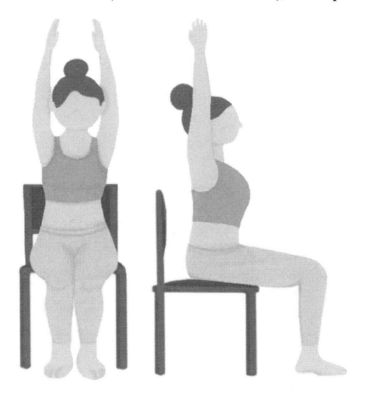

Step-by-Step Instructions:

- Sit up nice and tall in the chair toward the chair edge, so you aren't tempted to lean on the chair back.

- Keep your back straight, spine lengthened, and feet flat and firmly planted on the floor hip-width apart.

- Place your hands on your thighs with palms facing down.

- Drop your hands to the sides, then inhale as you raise both arms toward the ceiling.

- Hold here for 1–2 seconds, then exhale as you bring your arms back to your sides in a gentle and controlled manner.

- Repeat 10 times, breathing deeply each time.

3. Chair Relaxation Pose (Chair Savasana), 10 Deep Breaths

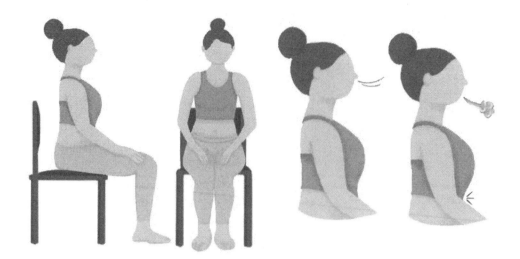

Step-by-Step Instructions:

- Sit up nice and tall in the chair, leaving some space behind you.

- Keep your back straight, spine lengthened, knees bent at a 90-degree angle, and feet flat and firmly planted on the floor hip-width apart.

- Place your hands on your thighs with your palms facing down.

- Keep your shoulders neutral, chest raised, and relax your limbs and face.

- Engage your abdomen slightly and pull your belly button toward your spine and up just a bit.

- Roll your shoulder blades down toward your back and relax your elbows at the sides.

- Now close your eyes and start breathing in and out deeply through your nose. Pay attention to your breathing to be sure it feels comfortable.

- Continue with this breathing for 10 deep breaths or set a timer for 30 seconds.

- Slowly and gently open your eyes and release your hands down by your sides to come out of the pose.

If you get to the end and have more time, you can do some more deep breathing. Feeling ready to jump into your new yoga routine? Commit to one 10-minute practice today and see how good you feel afterward.

Under 10-Minute Sequence at a Glance

For easy reference during your chair yoga practice session, here is a chart with images of all the poses described in this chapter at a glance:

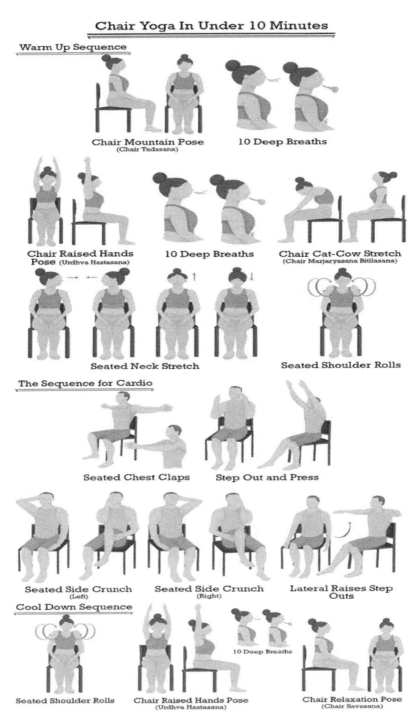

Chair Yoga In Under 10 Minutes

Warm Up Sequence

Chair Mountain Pose
(Chair Tadasana)

10 Deep Breaths

Chair Raised Hands Pose (Urdhva Hastasana)

10 Deep Breaths

Chair Cat-Cow Stretch
(Chair Marjaryasana Bitilasana)

Seated Neck Stretch

Seated Shoulder Rolls

The Sequence for Cardio

Seated Chest Claps

Step Out and Press

Seated Side Crunch
(Left)

Seated Side Crunch
(Right)

Lateral Raises Step Outs

Cool Down Sequence

Seated Shoulder Rolls

Chair Raised Hands Pose
(Urdhva Hastasana)

10 Deep Breaths

Chair Relaxation Pose
(Chair Savasana)

Chapter Seven:

The Best Diet for Weight Loss, Flexibility and Decreasing Inflammation

When it comes to wellness, physical exercise occupies a part of the equation, and nutrition and mindset occupy the remaining parts of the equation. The three factors together form a wellness triangle. Since we have already addressed two of these factors, we will now give nutrition the spotlight.

Exercise and nutrition work together to give you a healthy, strong body. While exercise provides the correct stimulus for muscle growth, nutrition provides your body with the energy required to fuel it. Working on your mindset rounds this out by keeping you motivated and excited to stay on track. Also, the less mental stress you have, the easier it is for your body to shed those pounds!

As mentioned earlier, weight loss or weight gain is largely determined by the number of calories you consume. When we mention calorie consumption, we are simply referring to your diet.

Your body doesn't need much to become strong, flexible, and healthy. It just needs a little lubrication, correct stimulus, and proper nutrients. It doesn't need a lot of analytical thinking or a degree in nutrition. In this concluding chapter, we're going to look at the simple dietary changes you can make in order to improve your body. Making healthy food decisions fuels your body and your mind and is easier to do than you might think.

Let's begin with dietary choices for flexibility improvement. We know how important flexibility and balance are to everyone. If your joints and other body parts aren't flexible, you won't be able to move. To keep your independence, you need to keep your flexibility and balance.

If any of your body parts can't complete their motion, that is a sign that you are not flexible. Although some people have a better range of motion than others, depending on their anatomy, other factors influence flexibility, including lifestyle and age.

Chair yoga is a good way to increase your body's flexibility, and here are some of the flexibility-enhancing foods to add to your diet that will make you become bendy and limber in no time!

Proteins

Protein is a very important nutrient to your body. It is the building block of all the muscles in your body. It helps repair, rebuild, and maintain your body tissues. Being the most satiating nutrient, protein can also contribute to weight loss because it makes you feel full faster and longer, which helps you consume fewer calories. In addition to this, it is not easy for a protein to be converted to stored fat like other macronutrients; this is due to its nitrogen content. Instead, your body stores the excess protein in your muscle tissues, which is then used later when your body is in high demand of protein, like during or after exercise. This helps reduce excess fat storage, resulting in weight loss. All these factors affect your flexibility because if your body fails to build some muscles, then you will become weak. And if you become overweight, then your flexibility is likely to suffer too.

Proteins also play other roles in your body, including regulation of body pH, protection against diseases, maintaining body water balance, transportation of oxygen, vitamins, minerals, biological processes, and coordination, among others. Just from this list, you can tell how important protein is to your body and imagine what could happen to you if you didn't have enough protein in your body. This clearly indicates that your body not only needs proteins to build and repair your muscles to make you strong and flexible, but it also needs protein to survive! Therefore, in order to build muscle mass and improve flexibility, you need to consume enough proteins. If you consume fewer proteins than you require, you risk losing muscle mass and flexibility.

The FDA recommends that an average person who just needs proteins to survive should consume 0.8 grams of protein per kilogram of their body weight (0.8 g/kg/d) or 0.36 grams per pound of their body weight (0.36 g/lb/d) on a daily basis. However, this recommendation is a bit low if you want to build muscle and improve body flexibility through exercise.

The highest amount of proteins your body can use in a day is 1.6 grams per kilogram of body weight or 0.73 grams per pound of body weight. However, to ensure that you get enough amino acids and make up for inaccuracy and variation, a buffer is added to the upper number (Morton et al., 2017). Therefore, the recommended amount of your daily protein intake is 1.8 grams per kilogram of your body weight; or 0.82 grams per pound of your body weight (Philips & van Loon, 2011). Consider increasing this by 10% if you are a vegan or a vegetarian.

Here are Some Sources of Proteins

Animal protein: fish, chicken, turkey, shellfish, eggs, beef, pork, lamb.

Plant protein: tofu, edamame (whole green soybean pods), nuts and seeds, plant-based. protein powder, beans and legumes (like lentils)

Try to choose organic proteins when possible, especially meat and soy products. This is even more important than choosing organic vegetables. If it is very expensive to do so in your area, cut back on buying unnecessary sweets and processed junk food to help with the cost. We will also touch on why it is helpful to cut these out later in the chapter.

Water/Hydration

Water constitutes a more significant percentage of your body mass than any other substance. About 80% of your body content is water, followed by proteins. This clearly indicates how important water is to your body. Water helps lubricate your joints and muscles, making them more flexible for movement. If your joints aren't lubricated, you won't take a single step or stretch. Your joints and muscles have to be elastic for any movement to occur. And proper hydration is what is needed.

If you fail to properly hydrate your body, you risk losing strength and muscular endurance. When you are dehydrated, you feel fatigued and too lazy to do anything. This means you won't be able to perform even the easiest yoga pose. You need to drink plenty of water if you want to avoid dehydration and be effective in your yoga routines. It is just as simple as that.

It is simple to add water to your diet and boost flexibility. Hydrate your body before, during, and after your yoga sessions if you want to perform your best and recover properly.

To easily add more water to your life, consider drinking a glass of water of at least 8 ounces with every meal, 8 ounces each time you take supplements, and 8 ounces each before, during, and after your yoga sessions or any other exercise session. This will help you hit your daily water intake recommendation of 2–3 quarts, make you feel fuller, and prevent you from getting extra calories that you might normally consume with another drink like fruit juice, soda, or alcohol. Another trick I have used is to start my day by filling up 3 quart-sized mason jars with filtered water and just keep drinking through them all day until they are gone. That way, I can see how close to my goal I am getting! You can also use a plastic pitcher with measurement lines on it.

You also can add high water content foods like broccoli, green cabbage, cauliflower, eggplant, and other vegetables to your diet to boost your hydration.

Green leafy vegetables

To flush out acids from your body, you need to consume foods with cleansing capabilities, such as green leafy vegetables. This also helps improve your flexibility. Such vegetables include: kale, spinach, chard, seaweed, collard greens, and watercress. Vegetables are also rich in fiber. Fiber has the fewest calories, thus lowering the energy density of the food. It also helps improve metabolism by slowing down the rate at which food is digested, increasing the thermal effect of food. Fiber also enhances satiation because it stimulates chewing. Altogether, the mentioned benefits of fiber help with weight loss. Remember, being overweight can also affect flexibility.

Barley grass

Barley grass contains beta-carotene, iron, and high levels of calcium. All these improve your overall health and increase your flexibility. Calcium is the primary building block of bones. And strong bones equate to flexibility. The calcium in barley grass can also help prevent or reverse osteoporosis.

Barley grass is also a nutritious vegetable with a lot of fiber. The fiber helps improve metabolism as well as enhance satiation, which in turn helps with weight loss.

Blending it into your morning smoothie can really help increase your flexibility. But be warned that it will turn your smoothie bright green. You could alternatively take barley grass tablets. I personally think it makes the smoothie look cool, but it's not for everyone!

Spirulina

This is an algae with a great number of essential vitamins such as B complex and beta-carotene, both of which are very important in boosting muscle strength. Spirulina also lets you stretch with ease because it keeps muscle cramps at bay. It also can be added to smoothies; same note as above that it will turn your smoothies bright green and can be taken in tablet form. You can also find combination powders and tablets with spirulina and barley grass in them.

Sulfur

After calcium and phosphorus, sulfur is the third most abundant mineral in your body. Methionine and cysteine are the two amino acids used to make proteins and contain sulfur. Sulfur helps protect your body cells and tissues from damage and helps keep them strong and flexible. Sulfur also improves your metabolism, thus aiding digestion, which, in turn, contributes to healthy skin, tendons, and ligaments. Foods rich in sulfur include: garlic, onions, egg yolks, red peppers, and cruciferous vegetables such as kale, bok choy, cauliflower, and broccoli.

Amino acids

Your body requires certain amino acids in order to repair damaged connective tissues and regenerate healthy ones. Foods rich in amino acids promote flexible muscles, tendons, ligaments, and joints and give elasticity to the skin. Glycine, hydroxyproline, proline, and alanine are the best amino acids to target if you need to improve flexibility and recovery. These amino acids are found in foods like fish, poultry, and meat. If you can't get enough of them from your diet, consider consuming them in the form of supplements.

Foods rich in collagen

Collagen is the most abundant protein in your body, taking up a third of all your body proteins and three-quarters of your skin. It is also the main protein from which connective tissues are made. Connective tissues are all over your body. They make up several parts of your body, including bones, tendons, ligaments, muscles, and skin. Collagen is known for promoting healthy joints and adding elasticity to the skin. Consuming foods that are rich in collagen helps strengthen your bones, thus improving flexibility. As you grow older, your body collagen lessens. That's why it is important to boost it by consuming collagen-rich foods. Foods that are rich in collagen include:

- Vitamin C-rich foods like oranges and other citrus fruits

- Broccoli, Brussels sprouts, and cauliflower

- Green and red peppers

- Spinach, cabbage, and other leafy greens

Foods for Decreasing Inflammation in the Joints

Inflammation can become problematic when it's low-grade and chronic. Research shows that what you eat can affect the levels of C-reactive protein (CRP), which is a marker for inflammation. Some foods release inflammatory messengers, while others help your body fight oxidative stress. Here are some good diet choices for decreasing inflammation:

Eat more whole plant foods

Your body is more likely to burn more calories through digestion when you eat whole plant foods than processed ones. Processed foods are easier to break down during digestion than whole foods. It takes a lot of effort to break down whole food—right from chewing to the actual digestion. This process increases the Thermic Effect of Food (TEF), which refers to the number of calories burned through digestion.

Besides increasing the TEF, whole plant foods are also rich in fiber. Fiber is very helpful in that it offers great satiation. It makes you feel full faster, thus decreasing hunger feelings and preventing overeating. In other words, whole plant foods keep you fuller for longer and burn more calories during digestion which in turn helps with fat loss. That is a win-win for improved flexibility and reduced inflammation because excess fat gain can make you less flexible and clog your blood vessels, preventing the smooth flow of blood and other body liquids and causing inflammation.

Most plant-based foods are also good sources of antioxidants. Antioxidants help prevent or slow down cell damage that may be caused by unstable molecules that your body produces in reaction to the environment and other pressures. Whole plant foods include: tomatoes, kale, spinach, collard greens, bell peppers, mushrooms, etc.

Get Omega-3 fatty acids

Essential fatty acids are very important to our health and well-being. Since our body doesn't produce these fatty acids, the only way to ensure that our body gets them is by adding them to the meals we consume. Alpha-linolenic acid (ALA) and linolenic acid (LA) are the two main essential fatty acids. Your body gets omega-6 fatty acids from ALA and omega-3 fatty acids from LA. Oily fish like sardines, mackerel, and salmon are great sources of these fatty acids.

An abundance of research shows that both omega-3 and omega-6 fatty acids have tremendous health benefits to your body. One study conducted on the inflammatory effects of both fatty acids showed that while omega-3 fatty acid is anti-inflammatory, omega-6 fatty acid decreases the risk of heart disease (Johnson & Fritsche, 2012).

Therefore, to prevent inflammation, it is recommended that you consume enough omega-3 fatty acids. Besides omega-3s being anti-inflammatory, they also bestow on your body the following health benefits:

- Enhance body fat loss and prevent you from gaining more excess body fat.
- Lower your cortisol levels, thus contributing to improved moods and reduced depression (Wani et al., 2015).
- Increase cognitive performance.
- Prevention of excessive muscle loss and damage (Huang et al., 2020).
- Better insulin sensitivity (Black et al., 2018).
- Reduce muscle and joint soreness.
- And much more!

Consume Healthy Fats

The food we consume has two types of fat: triglycerides and cholesterol. In most cases, we consume triglycerides found in foods like avocados, olive oil, meat, fish, nuts, etc. So triglycerides and fatty acids are the major components of nutritional fats.

Triglycerides are then divided into two types: saturated and unsaturated. Saturated triglycerides contain all the hydrogen atoms and are mostly solid at room temperature. Unsaturated triglycerides, also known as unsaturated fats, lack at least one hydrogen atom and are mostly liquid at room temperature. They have many health benefits, including the absorption of vitamins A, D, E, and K, promoting healthy hair and skin, hormone development, and reduced inflammation, among others. That is why they are referred to as "healthy fats" or "good fats." So when we mention healthy fats, we are simply referring to unsaturated fats, which are found in foods like olives, avocados, fish, sesame seeds, almonds, walnuts, and other nuts.

The anti-inflammatory property of unsaturated fats comes in due to its oily nature at room temperature. The fact that it is liquid at room temperature means that they are less likely to eventually gunk up your arteries, causing blockage of blood and liquid flow.

The fat-free/low-fat craze of the 80s really caused a lot of health problems when people started cutting out these healthy fats. It's crucial to know the difference between good healthy fats, which have been referenced above, and unhealthy fats, which we will cover later in this chapter.

Take Green Tea

You may have heard that green tea is a healthy beverage to drink. Multiple studies have found that there is an association between green tea consumption and reduced risk of chronic conditions (Molina et al., 2015).

Green tea has a catechin or, rather, a substance called epigallocatechin-3-gallate (EGCG), which gives it antioxidant and anti-inflammatory properties, thus the above health benefits. EGCG helps prevent or lower the production of pro-inflammatory cytokines as well as prevent damage to fatty acid cells in your body, thus inhibiting inflammation (Eng et al., 2018). Be aware that it does contain a little caffeine (so does dark chocolate and cocoa listed next). So it's better for some people to consume these earlier in the day.

Enjoy Dark Chocolate and Cocoa

Who doesn't like chocolate? Besides dark chocolate being delicious and satisfying, it also has antioxidants that help reduce inflammation. It has cocoa flavanols, which give it anti-inflammatory properties and help keep the endothelial cells lining your arteries healthy.

This helps prevent and reduce the risks of heart disease and other age-related conditions (Khan et al., 2014).

A study conducted on healthy young and elderly people showed that those who consumed 700 mg of cocoa flavanols daily for two weeks experienced improved vascular function (Grone et al., 2019). Be aware that, like green tea, it does contain a little caffeine, so it's better for some people to consume these earlier in the day. But other than that disclaimer, go get that dark chocolate and enjoy!

Add Turmeric to Your Diet

Turmeric contains curcumin, which gives it its powerful anti-inflammatory properties (Nabavi et al., 2015). This helps reduce inflammation that may be caused by arthritis, diabetes, and other related conditions (Pivari et al., 2019).

A study conducted on people with metabolic syndrome who consumed a gram of curcumin every day showed that they experienced a significant reduction in the inflammatory marker CRP (Hewlings & Kalman, 2017).

Consume Ginger

Ginger isn't just delicious. Its health benefits are amazing. Ginger has a bioactive compound called gingerol, which gives it its anti-inflammatory, antioxidant, and many other medicinal properties. Gingerol also has a stimulating effect on the circulatory system. This makes it one of the most important foods or spices to add to your diet. Research shows that ginger helps reduce oxidative stress, thus preventing damage to body cells, ligaments, tendons, and inflammation by reducing the number of free radicals in the body (Wang et al., 2014). Due to its anti-inflammatory nature, ginger can also help treat arthritis.

Foods to Limit or Cut Out Completely!

If you want to lose weight, become more flexible, and prevent inflammation, here are the foods you need to cut out from your diet completely or limit their consumption:

Refined Carbohydrates

Refined carbohydrates refer to carbohydrates that have been processed and stripped of all the fiber, bran, and some nutrients. As much as your body requires carbs to provide energy for fueling your daily activities, it is very important to choose carbohydrates that are good for your health. You are advised to go for complex carbohydrates and avoid simple or refined carbohydrates. Let me explain why.

Most complex carbs have fiber in them. As mentioned earlier, fiber is satiating (it makes you feel full faster and longer) when consumed. This helps prevent you from feeling hungry, thus eating less, which, in turn, leads to weight loss. Complex carbs also take more time to digest. This increases the Thermic Effect of Food (TEF), which boosts your metabolism. This helps you burn more calories during digestion.

Refined carbs, on the other hand, lack fiber and nutrients. They tend to also contain added sugars which makes them have the poorest satiety and nutritional value. Sugar doesn't make you full. When you consume any food with added sugar, you always want to eat more. This makes you overeat, thus leading to weight gain.

Refined carbs are also easy to digest. This gives them the lowest TEF. This means that your metabolism is affected, which results in burning fewer calories during digestion or no calories at all. This is another way refined carbs can result in weight gain!

Consuming a lot of refined carbs also floods your bloodstream with sugar. This triggers a surge of insulin to clear sugar from your blood. And with time, this can lead to insulin resistance and type 2 diabetes. Refined carbs are present in foods like white bread, white pasta, pizza, white rice, sweet desserts, breakfast cereals, cakes, and many other baked foods. But luckily, there are many better alternatives these days: unrefined whole grains, such as whole wheat or multigrain bread and pasta, brown rice, quinoa, oatmeal, brown rice flour or cauliflower pizza crust, whole wheat flour, and brown rice flour can be used in baked goods instead of refined white flour. Also, starchy vegetables such as sweet potatoes, red potatoes, squashes such as butternut squash and acorn squash, corn, rice cauliflower, and legumes can make wonderful substitutes. And these last suggestions are whole plant food complex carbohydrates! People who follow the popular and successful Paleo and Keto diets only eat whole food, plant-based complex carbohydrates in addition to proteins and healthy fats—and that is one of the reasons they are so effective in achieving weight loss.

Sugar

When starting on a weight loss and inflammation reduction program, one of the most powerful things you can do is to avoid anything with added sugars at all costs. Sugar is one of the worst offenders on this list when it comes to contributing to weight gain and inflammation, and it can lead to a host of other health problems as well. Consuming too many sugars increase the inflammatory markers in your blood. Remember, it is very easy to overconsume sugar once you start consuming it due to its poor satiation. Several studies have associated dietary sugar consumption with chronic inflammation. A meta-analysis of several interventional studies conducted on the effects of dietary sugar intake on biomarkers of inflammation indicated that dietary sugar consumption contributes to increased inflammatory processes in humans (Della Corte et al., 2018).

Another study conducted on the links between added sugar and inflammation showed that consuming sweetened drinks impairs glucose and lipid metabolism and promotes inflammation. The study included 29 healthy people who consumed a 375 ml can of soda with only 40 grams of added sugar every day. After three weeks, the participants experienced increased inflammation, insulin resistance, and LDL cholesterol (Aeberli et al., 2011). So to lose weight and avoid chronic inflammation and the associated diseases, limit or avoid foods and substances with added sugars like sweetened drinks such as soda and other beverages, sugary snacks, etc. Read labels and watch out for white refined sugar, high fructose corn syrup, and even brown sugar. Replace these with natural, unprocessed, unrefined sugars such as stevia, coconut sugar, or agave nectar. Also, look for better sweet treats like fruit, coconut water, tea sweetened with stevia, baked goods with coconut sugar, ice creams sweetened with agave nectar or coconut sugar, and chocolate sweetened with stevia or coconut sugar.

Margarine and Shortening

These are saturated fats commonly touted as "bad fats." As mentioned earlier, saturated fats are solid at room temperature and are less satiating as compared to unsaturated fats. This means that you are more likely to overeat saturated fat than unsaturated fats. This overeating can result in weight gain. Fats are calorie dense. They have more calories than other macronutrients like carbs and proteins. Therefore, consuming them in surplus increases the number of calories in no time, which could lead to obesity.

Junk Foods and Processed Meats

Junk foods and processed meats are dangerously high in sodium, nitrate, and unhealthy fats. These preservatives may cause arteries to stiffen to prevent the smooth flow of blood and other body fluids, thus causing inflammation. Excess sodium also dehydrates your body because it pulls all the liquid from your body cells. As a result, your body tries to hold on to fluids in order to dilute the blood. This leads to swollen joints and other body parts.

Weight Loss, Anti-Inflammatory, and Flexibility Diet Tips

- When doing your weekly shopping, fill your shopping cart with a variety of proteins, starchy vegetables, and other vegetables. Shop around the outside perimeter of the store—that is where the produce section, the meat section, and the seafood sections are. Essentially where all the whole foods are. The inner aisles are filled with processed and packaged foods.

- Replace fast foods with healthy whole food choices.

- Replace sugary beverages and drinks with sparkling mineral water, coconut water, filtered water with cucumber slices and lemon slices, and hot/iced tea sweetened with stevia.

- Eat meals that consist of mostly whole foods, giving you a variety of vitamins and minerals.

- Read labels: Avoid unhealthy fats, refined sugars, refined carbohydrates, and processed packaged foods with preservatives and additives.

- Eat healthy fats: Put olive oil on salads, cook with avocado oil, and eat nuts, seeds, olives, and avocados. Consume omega-3 fatty acids like salmon, sardines, cod liver oil (good on salads), flax seeds, and walnuts.

- The majority of your food intake should be whole foods, not processed.

- Form a sustainable meal plan consisting of all the healthy foods discussed in this chapter. Use a shopping list to stick to the plan. Or have groceries delivered so you're not tempted to impulse buy, and you also save gas that way! Create two weekly menus and rotate through both of them for variety.

As you take the next step into your health journey, you'll find yourself feeling healthier, happier, and even younger. Congratulations on making this choice for your future!

Conclusion

The numerous health benefits of yoga practice cannot be overemphasized, regardless of your age, gender, and other factors. It is never too late to get moving, release stress, and stretch every joint and muscle in your body while reaping all the benefits that come with it. The infamous muscle loss, weight gain, lack of flexibility, and imbalance among seniors worsen when you remain physically inactive. Don't allow aching joints and stubborn fat buildup to bother you anymore. You can get rid of them without having to strain too much. You can enjoy all the health benefits of yoga without having to get up and down off of the floor or stressing your joints. Performing yoga in a chair is a safe and gentle answer.

You may have overheard some of the false information about yoga and avoided practicing yoga at all costs. There is no time like the present to get started!

It might not be that simple to start practicing yoga and stay consistent right away if you haven't been doing it. You may experience some challenges, disappointments, and frustrations. Cut yourself some slack, be compassionate with yourself, and keep going! Remember, adaptation is a gradual process; it doesn't happen overnight. It demands changes in your lifestyle, routine, and ways of doing things. And with the right mindset and attitude, everything will fall into place. Never underestimate the power of your mind and having a growth mindset. Develop your mind's resilience and build the tenacity to triumph over any challenge and obstacles that come your way.

As you practice your chair yoga exercise, remember to consume a healthy diet, and keep your mindset strong for optimum results. Diet, mindset, and exercise act as the pillars for building the foundation of a structure, which in this case is your health. They all contribute to your wellness triangle.

Get support and help to stay on track. Facebook groups, community centers, senior centers, accountability buddies, and wellness-minded friends and family can all help you stay focused on achieving your health goals. Find encouraging and supportive people to surround yourself with who will cheer you on and who you can lean on when you need to. Don't underestimate the power of having a supportive community around you to help you become the best you that you can be!

Key Takeaways

- Yoga is more than just a physical form of exercise—it's a spiritual, mindful practice with a host of benefits.

- You can reap all the benefits of yoga by practicing it in the chair.

- Always seek your doctor's advice and get the green light before participating in yoga if you have any medical conditions or injuries.

- Practicing yoga can help relieve stress and depression.

- You can eliminate stubborn fat buildup through yoga poses and cardio movements.

- The breathing techniques in yoga practice help with respiration and relaxation.

- Yoga enhances flexibility, mobility, balance, and stability.

- Yoga is also helpful in chronic disease management, body strengthening, improved mental health, and the mind-body connection.

- You don't have to be super flexible in order to begin your yoga practice.

- Yoga poses engage muscles that you don't normally use, which adds a different element to your workout and offers you a variety of movements.

- Age is not a determining factor for physical activity; it is never too late to start yoga.

- Adaptation is a gradual process, and it demands a change of routine to achieve this. You need to assess your mindset and let go of any limiting beliefs.

- Always start your exercises with warm-ups. It helps reduce the risks of injuries, thus enhancing your performance.

- Cooldowns give your mind time to settle into the calming experience of yoga and recover.

- Pair your yoga practice with a healthy diet if you want to achieve your optimal weight loss goals.

- Stay properly hydrated to enhance your yoga practice performance and increase flexibility. Drink enough water daily and consume foods with high water content and fiber, such as fruits, starchy vegetables, and vegetables.

- Above all, consistency is key. Make your chair yoga practice a habit and stick with it.

Congratulations, you have come to the end of this book! Now you have all it takes to stay strong, flexible, balanced, happier, and healthier. The information in this book will be powerless to change your health, body, and life if you don't take action. Begin by making one healthful choice for yourself this week and see the changes start to happen!

My hope is that you will find the poses, programs, and better food choices in this book helpful and quickly start reaping the amazing benefits that wellness living has to offer. Regaining your health gives you back the ability to enjoy yourself and have the energy for the most important things in your life! I hope that yoga practice and movement will become something you enjoy and make you happy. I wish you good luck on this amazing journey that will grant you an opportunity for a thriving, joyful, and more purposeful life in your golden years!

If you enjoyed reading this book or learned something from it, please leave me a review on Amazon. Each review helps me spread these messages to more people.

Thank you from the bottom of my heart!

A FREE GIFT TO ALL MY READERS!

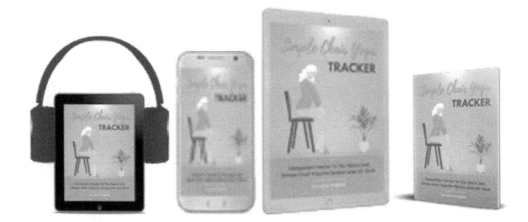

Dear Friends,

As a thank you and to help you stay dedicated to stick to your chair yoga and exercise goals, I would like to send you a free copy of my colorful 30-day simple chair yoga tracker so you can track your progress at home and keep your motivation alive!

To get your free copy now, please visit:

www.gesundbooks.com

References

Aeberli, I., Gerber, P. A., Hochuli, M., Kohler, S., Haile, S. R., Gouni-Berthold, I., Berthold, H. K., Spinas, G. A., & Berneis, K. (2011). *Low to moderate sugar-sweetened beverage consumption impairs glucose and lipid metabolism and promotes inflammation in healthy young men*: a randomized controlled trial. The American Journal of Clinical Nutrition, 94(2), 479–485. https://doi.org/10.3945/ajcn.111.013540.

Aerobic exercise: *How to warm up and cool down.* (2021, October 6). Mayo Clinic. https://www.mayoclinic.org/healthy-lifestyle/fitness/in-depth/exercise/art-20045517?reDate=29082022.

American Diabetes Association | *Research, Education, Advocacy.* (n.d.). American Diabetes Association. https://www.diabetes.org.

Anderer, J. (2021, September 29). *Over 60? These 5 walking tips will help you lose weight.* Eat This Not That. https://www.eatthis.com/news-steps-walking-lose-weight-after-60/.

Bird, S. R., & Hawley, J. A. (2017). *Update on the effects of physical activity on insulin sensitivity in humans.* BMJ Open Sport & Exercise Medicine, 2(1), e000143. https://doi.org/10.1136/bmjsem-2016-000143.

Boggenpoel, E. (2021, October 7). *6 yoga myths debunked.* Livescience.com. https://www.livescience.com/6-yoga-myths-debunked.

Bouschet, C. L. (2020, February 28). *How to add a yoga practice into your routine.* Life Goals Mag. https://lifegoalsmag.com/how-to-add-a-yoga-practice-into-your-routine/.

Byzak, A. (2018, December 29). *Why warming up and cooling down is important.* Tri-City Medical Center. https://www.tricitymed.org/2016/12/warming-cooling-important/.

Calories burned during exercise, activities, sports and workouts. (n.d.). NUTRISTRATEGY. http://www.nutristrategy.com/caloriesburned.htm.

Center, T. G. (2022, March 9). *10 day chair workout to lose belly fat (no standing).* YouTube. https://www.youtube.com/watch?v=g0jru_yb7dk&feature=youtu.be.

Chang, D. G., & Kertesz, S. G. (2017). *Yoga and low back pain: no fool's tool.* Annals of Internal Medicine, 167(2), 129. https://doi.org/10.7326/m17-1263.

Chaten. (2017, August 16). *Unmotivated? Remind yourself of your reason why.* ConnecTeen. https://calgaryconnecteen.com/find-your-reasons/.

Crowley, K. (2020, November 22). *Struggling to loosen up your limbs? 7 foods to improve your flexibility.* Gymondo® Magazine: Fitness, Nutrition & Weight Loss. https://www.gymondo.com/magazin/en/nutrition-en/struggling-to-loosen-up-your-limbs-7-foods-to-improve-your-flexibility.

Csala, B. (2021). *The relationship between yoga and spirituality:* A systematic review of empirical research. Frontiers. https://www.frontiersin.org/articles/10.3389/fpsyg.2021.695939/full.

Della Corte, K., Perrar, I., Penczynski, K., Schwingshackl, L., Herder, C., & Buyken, A. (2018). *Effect of dietary sugar intake on biomarkers of subclinical inflammation:* A systematic review and meta-analysis of intervention studies. Nutrients, 10(5), 606. https://doi.org/10.3390/nu10050606.

Derrick. (2021a, July 6). *Chair yoga for seniors - 17 great stretches.* Elder Guru. https://www.elderguru.com/chair-yoga-for-seniors-17-great-stretches/.

Dhikav, V., Karmarkar, G., Verma, M., Gupta, R., Gupta, S., Mittal, D., & Anand, K. (2010). Y*oga in male sexual functioning: A noncomparative pilot study.* The Journal of Sexual Medicine, 7(10), 3460–3466. https://doi.org/10.1111/j.1743-6109.2010.01930.x.

Domonell, K. D. B. (2016, January 13). *Why endorphins (and exercise) make you happy.* CNN. https://edition.cnn.com/2016/01/13/health/endorphins-exercise-cause-happiness/.

Eng, Q. Y., Thanikachalam, P. V., & Ramamurthy, S. (2018). *Molecular understanding of Epigallocatechin gallate (EGCG) in cardiovascular and metabolic diseases.* Journal of Ethnopharmacology, 210, 296–310. https://doi.org/10.1016/j.jep.2017.08.035.

Gopinath, B., Kifley, A., Flood, V. M., & Mitchell, P. (2018). *Physical activity as a determinant of successful aging over ten years.* Scientific Reports, 8(1). https://doi.org/10.1038/s41598-018-28526-3.

Grabara, M., & Szopa, J. (2015). *Effects of hatha yoga exercises on spine flexibility in women over 50 years old.* Journal of Physical Therapy Science, 27(2), 361–365. https://doi.org/10.1589/jpts.27.361.

Gröne, M., Sansone, R., Höffken, P., Horn, P., Rodriguez-Mateos, A., Schroeter, H., Kelm, M., & Heiss, C. (2019). *Cocoa flavanols improve endothelial functional integrity in healthy young and elderly subjects.* Journal of Agricultural and Food Chemistry, 68(7), 1871–1876. https://doi.org/10.1021/acs.jafc.9b02251.

Gwinup, G. (1987). *Weight loss without dietary restriction: Efficacy of different forms of aerobic exercise.* The American Journal of Sports Medicine, 15(3), 275–279. https://doi.org/10.1177/036354658701500317.

Harris, M. L. (2019, January 31). *The truth is stunning: No age limits for marathon runners.* Sixty and Me. https://sixtyandme.com/the-truth-is-stunning-no-age-limits-for-marathon-runners/

Harvard Health Publishing. (2018, November 7). Foods that fight inflammation - Harvard Health. Harvard Health; Harvard Health. https://www.health.harvard.edu/staying-healthy/foods-that-fight-inflammation

Hewlings, S., & Kalman, D. (2017). Curcumin: A review of its effects on human health. Foods, 6(10), 92. https://doi.org/10.3390/foods6100092.

How to use food to help your body fight inflammation. (2019, August 13). Mayo Clinic. https://www.mayoclinic.org/healthy-lifestyle/nutrition-and-healthy-eating/in-depth/how-to-use-food-to-help-your-body-fight-inflammation/art-20457586?reDate=29082022.

Huang, Y. H., Chiu, W. C., Hsu, Y. P., Lo, Y. L., & Wang, Y. H. (2020). *Effects of omega-3 fatty acids on muscle mass, muscle strength and muscle performance among the elderly: A meta-analysis.* Nutrients, 12(12), 3739. DOI: 10.3390/nu12123739.

Johnson, G. H., & Fritsche, K. (2012). *Effect of dietary linoleic acid on markers of inflammation in healthy persons: A systematic review of randomized controlled trials.* Journal of the Academy of Nutrition and Dietetics, 112(7), 1029–1041.e15. https://doi.org/10.1016/j.jand.2012.03.029.

Jordan, C. (2019, November 25). *Chair cardio for fat loss: Seated no impact fitness class*. YouTube. https://www.youtube.com/watch?v=_nZ07OVtSmQ&feature=youtu.be.

Kanaya, A. M., Araneta, M. R. G., Pawlowsky, S. B., Barrett-Connor, E., Grady, D., Vittinghoff, E., Schembri, M., Chang, A., Carrion-Petersen, M. L., Coggins, T., Tanori, D., Armas, J. M., & Cole, R. J. (2014). *Restorative yoga and metabolic risk factors: The practicing restorative yoga vs. stretching for the metabolic syndrome (PRYSMS) randomized trial*. Journal of Diabetes and Its Complications, 28(3), 406–412. https://doi.org/10.1016/j.jdiacomp.2013.12.001.

Khalsa, S. B. S. (2004). Treatment of chronic insomnia with yoga: A preliminary study with sleep? Wake diaries. Applied Psychophysiology and Biofeedback, 29(4), 269–278. https://doi.org/10.1007/s10484-004-0387-0.

Khan, N., Khymenets, O., Urpí-Sardà, M., Tulipani, S., Garcia-Aloy, M., Monagas, M., Mora-Cubillos, X., Llorach, R., & Andres-Lacueva, C. (2014). *Cocoa polyphenols and inflammatory markers of cardiovascular disease*. Nutrients, 6(2), 844–880. https://doi.org/10.3390/nu6020844.

Kim, E. S., Hagan, K. A., Grodstein, F., DeMeo, D. L., de Vivo, I., & Kubzansky, L. D. (2016). *Optimism and cause-specific mortality: A prospective cohort study*. American Journal of Epidemiology, 185(1), 21–29. https://doi.org/10.1093/aje/kww182.

Lam, H. K. N., Middleton, H., & Phillips, S. M. (2021). *The effect of self-selected music on endurance running capacity and performance in a mentally fatigued state*. Journal of Human Sport and Exercise, 17(4). https://doi.org/10.14198/jhse.2022.174.16.

Lauche, R., Langhorst, J., Lee, M. S., Dobos, G., & Cramer, H. (2016). *A systematic review and meta-analysis on the effects of yoga on weight-related outcomes*. Preventive Medicine, 87, 213–232. https://doi.org/10.1016/j.ypmed.2016.03.013.

Longwell, C. (2020, October 28). *5 benefits of exercise for seniors and aging adults*. The GreenFields Continuing Care Community. https://thegreenfields.org/5-benefits-exercise-seniors-aging-adults/.

Martin, R., Prichard, I., Hutchinson, A. D., & Wilson, C. (2013). *The role of body awareness and mindfulness in the relationship between exercise and eating behavior*. Journal of Sport and Exercise Psychology, 35(6), 655–660. https://doi.org/10.1123/jsep.35.6.655.

McClelland, K. (2021, February 9). *A guide to physical wellness for seniors*. Where You Live Matters: A Senior Living Resource. ASHA. https://www.whereyoulivematters.org/physical-wellness-for-seniors/.

Milly, H. (2020, January 29). *Lose hanging lower belly fat sitting - Beginner friendly chair workout | Hana Milly*. YouTube. https://www.youtube.com/watch?v=0x_MsUr3tag&feature=youtu.be.

Molina, N., Bolin, A., & Otton, R. (2015). *Green tea polyphenols change the profile of inflammatory cytokine release from lymphocytes of obese and lean rats and protect against oxidative damage*. International Immunopharmacology, 28(2), 985–996. https://doi.org/10.1016/j.intimp.2015.08.011.

Moore, C. P. (2022, August 21). 11 *Mindset activities and tests designed to nurture growth*. PositivePsychology.com. https://positivepsychology.com/mindset-activities-tests/.

Morton, R. W., Murphy, K. T., McKellar, S. R., Schoenfeld, B. J., Henselmans, M., Helms, E., Aragon, A. A., Devries, M. C., Banfield, L., Krieger, J. W., & Phillips, S. M. (2017). *A systematic review, meta-analysis and meta-regression of the effect of protein supplementation on resistance training-induced gains in muscle mass and strength in healthy adults*. British Journal of Sports Medicine, 52(6), 376–384. DOI: 10.1136/bjsports-2017-097608.

Nabavi, S., Thiagarajan, R., Rastrelli, L., Daglia, M., Sobarzo-Sanchez, E., Alinezhad, H., & Nabavi, S. (2015). *Curcumin: A natural product for diabetes and its complications*. Current Topics in Medicinal Chemistry, 15(23), 2445–2455. https://doi.org/10.2174/1568026615666150619142519.

Neumark-Sztainer, D., MacLehose, R. F., Watts, A. W., Pacanowski, C. R., & Eisenberg, M. E. (2018). *Yoga and body image: Findings from a large population-based study of young adults*. Body Image, 24, 69–75. https://doi.org/10.1016/j.bodyim.2017.12.003.

Older Adults | Surgeon general report | CDC. (1999, November 17). CDC.Gov. https://www.cdc.gov/nccdphp/sgr/olderad.htm.

Origym. (2022, March 22). *21 Yoga myths and misconceptions explained.* https://origympersonaltrainercourses.co.uk/blog/yoga-myths-explained.

Osei-Tutu, K. B., & Campagna, P. D. (2005). *The effects of short- vs. long-bout exercise on mood, VO2max., and percent body fat.* Preventive Medicine, 40(1), 92–98. https://doi.org/10.1016/j.ypmed.2004.05.005.

Pae, G., & Akar, G. (2020). *Effects of walking on self-assessed health status: Links between walking, trip purposes and health.* Journal of Transport & Health, 18, 100901. https://doi.org/10.1016/j.jth.2020.100901.

Palmer, A. (2022, May 24). Yoga for seniors. Senior Living & Nursing Homes in Indiana. https://www.asccare.com/yoga-for-seniors/.

Pascoe, M. C., Thompson, D. R., & Ski, C. F. (2017). *Yoga, mindfulness-based stress reduction and stress-related physiological measures:* A meta-analysis. Psychoneuroendocrinology, 86, 152–168. https://doi.org/10.1016/j.psyneuen.2017.08.008.

Phillips, S. M., & van Loon, L. J. (2011). *Dietary protein for athletes: From requirements to optimum adaptation.* Journal of Sports Sciences, 29(sup1), S29–S38. DOI: 10.1080/02640414.2011.619204.

Pivari, F., Mingione, A., Brasacchio, C., & Soldati, L. (2019). *Curcumin and Type 2 Diabetes Mellitus: prevention and treatment.* Nutrients, 11(8), 1837. https://doi.org/10.3390/nu11081837.

Pizer, A. (2020, February 26). *10 yoga poses you can do in a chair.* Verywell Fit. https://www.verywellfit.com/chair-yoga-poses-3567189.

Polsgrove, M., Eggleston, B., & Lockyer, R. (2016). *Impact of 10-weeks of yoga practice on flexibility and balance of college athletes.* International Journal of Yoga, 9(1), 27. https://doi.org/10.4103/0973-6131.171710.

Raquel. (2020, May 2). 9 Ways to Make Yoga a Daily Habit (that will stick). Prettyeasylife.com. https://www.prettyeasylife.com/9-ways-to-make-yoga-a-daily-habit-that-will-stick/

Ramos-Jiménez, A., Wall-Medrano, A., Corona-Hernández, R., & Hernández-Torres, R. (2015). *Yoga, bioenergetics and eating behaviors:* A conceptual review. International Journal of Yoga, 8(2), 89. https://doi.org/10.4103/0973-6131.158469.

Renner, B. (2022, March 30). *Dog owners walk 1,000 miles, play 2,080 games of fetch with Fido each year*. Study Finds. https://studyfinds.org/dog-owners-1000-miles-fetch-walking-dogs-study/.

Robinson, M. M., Dasari, S., Konopka, A. R., Johnson, M. L., Manjunatha, S., Esponda, R. R., Carter, R. E., Lanza, I. R., & Nair, K. S. (2017). *Enhanced protein translation underlies improved metabolic and physical adaptations to different exercise training modes in young and old humans*. Cell Metabolism, 25(3), 581–592. https://doi.org/10.1016/j.cmet.2017.02.009.

Santos-Longhurst, A. (2019, February 21). *Benefits of thinking positively, and how to do it*. Healthline. https://www.healthline.com/health/how-to-think-positive.

Staff, L. (2021, December 1). *The flexibility diet*. LEMAlab. https://www.lemalab.eu/blogs/journal/the-flexibility-diet.

More Life Health Seniors. (2019b, April 1). *Standing warm-up routine for seniors (do before undertaking exercise)*. YouTube. https://www.youtube.com/watch?v=b2DYU7ZQgN0.

Stoller, A. (2019, August 29). *Are you ever too old to run a marathon?* Aaptiv. https://aaptiv.com/magazine/too-old-running-marathons#:%7E:text=In%20other%20words%2C%20plenty%20of,%2C%20the%20number%20drops%20down.%E2%80%9D.

Stress relief from laughter? *It's no joke*. (2021, July 29). Mayo Clinic. https://www.mayoclinic.org/healthy-lifestyle/stress-management/in-depth/stress-relief/art-20044456.

support@sitecare.com. (2022, July 22). *Home – HelpGuide*. HelpGuide.Org. https://www.helpguide.org/laughter-is-the-best-medicine.

Tappenden, M. (2016, December 20). *Yoga and weight loss*. In:Spa Retreats. https://www.inspa-retreats.com/latest-news/weight-loss/yoga-and-weight-loss/.

Tilbrook, H. E., Cox, H., Hewitt, C. E., Kang'ombe, A. R., Chuang, L. H., Jayakody, S., Aplin, J. D., Semlyen, A., Trewhela, A., Watt, I., & Torgerson, D. J. (2011). *Yoga for chronic low back pain.* Annals of Internal Medicine, 155(9), 569. https://doi.org/10.7326/0003-4819-155-9-201111010-00003.

Wang, S., Zhang, C., Yang, G., & Yang, Y. (2014). *Biological properties of 6-Gingerol: A brief review.* Natural Product Communications, 9(7), 1934578X1400900. https://doi.org/10.1177/1934578x1400900736.

Wani, A. L., Bhat, S. A., & Ara, A. (2015). *Omega-3 fatty acids and the treatment of depression: a review of scientific evidence.* Integrati Medicine Research, 4(3), 132–141. DOI: 10.1016/j.imr.2015.07.003.

Wu, Y. T., Luben, R., & Jones, A. (2017). *Dog ownership supports the maintenance of physical activity during poor weather in older English adults:* cross-sectional results from the EPIC Norfolk cohort. Journal of Epidemiology and Community Health, 71(9), 905–911. https://doi.org/10.1136/jech-2017-208987.

Yanek, L. R. (2021, November 1). *The power of positive thinking. Johns Hopkins Medicine.* https://www.hopkinsmedicine.org/health/wellness-and-prevention/the-power-of-positive-thinking.

Yoga Journal. (2020, October 20). *Chair yoga: 3 variations of tree pose.* https://www.yogajournal.com/video/chair-yoga-tree-pose-variations/.

Garfield, S. (2020, March 3). *What are some inspirational quotes about learning or sharing knowledge?* Medium. https://stangarfield.medium.com/what-are-some-inspirational-quotes-about-learning-or-sharing-knowledge-856751bdea6c

Can You Help Me Spread the Word?

I'm passionate about the power of chair yoga… and by now, I'm sure you are too. Will you help me spread the word far and wide?

All you have to do is leave your honest opinion of this book on Amazon, and other people like you will find the guidance they need to get started on this incredible journey.

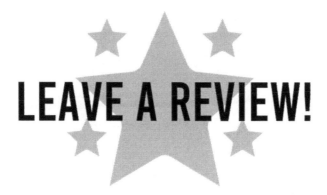

Let's help as many people as we can make those golden years shine. Thank you so much for helping me out here.

Made in the USA
Columbia, SC
26 August 2023

22131194R00083